PENGUIN BOOKS

THE OMEGA PRINCIPLE

Paul Greenberg is the author of the James Beard Award–winning bestseller *Four Fish* and *American Catch*, and is a regular contributor to *The New York Times*. His writing has also appeared in *The New Yorker*, *National Geographic*, and many other publications. A Pew Fellow in marine conservation and the Safina Center writer in residence, Greenberg has been a correspondent for PBS's *Frontline* and lectures widely on ocean issues at institutions ranging from TED to Google to the United States Senate. He lives in New York.

THE OMEGA PRINCIPLE

*Seafood and the Quest for a Long Life
and a Healthier Planet*

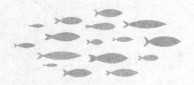

PAUL GREENBERG

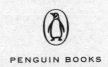

PENGUIN BOOKS

PENGUIN BOOKS
An imprint of Penguin Random House LLC
penguinrandomhouse.com

First published in the United States of America by Penguin Press,
an imprint of Penguin Random House LLC, 2018
Published in Penguin Books 2019

Portions of this book previously appeared in *The American Prospect*,
Eating Well magazine, and *Yale Environment 360*.

Image on page 148: Courtesy of Connecticut
Department of Energy & Environmental Protection
Images on page 179: NASA

ISBN 9780143111115 (paperback)

THE LIBRARY OF CONGRESS HAS CATALOGED THE
HARDCOVER EDITION AS FOLLOWS:
Names: Greenberg, Paul, 1967– author.
Title: The omega principle : seafood and the quest for a long life and a
healthier planet / Paul Greenberg.
Description: New York City : Penguin Press, 2018.
Identifiers: LCCN 2018006200 (print) | LCCN 2018010489 (ebook) |
ISBN 9780698183469 (ebook) | ISBN 9781594206344 (hardback)
Subjects: LCSH: Omega-3 fatty acids—Physiological effect. | Omega-3 fatty
acids—Therapeutic use. | BISAC: NATURE / Animals / Marine Life. |
COOKING / Specific Ingredients / Seafood. |
NATURE / Ecosystems & Habitats / Oceans & Seas.
Classification: LCC QP752.O44 (ebook) | LCC QP752.O44 G74 2018 (print) |
DDC 613.2/84—dc23
LC record available at https://lccn.loc.gov/2018006200

Printed in the United States of America
1 3 5 7 9 10 8 6 4 2

Designed by Amanda Dewey

For Tanya and Luke, essential supplements

It goes into your body and explodes inside into little stars that get into your blood and brush off all the bad things that get stuck on it. They massage your heart to make it work better and help your brain think smarter.

—*Omega-3 user survey*

CONTENTS

INTRODUCTION

On a recent July morning I stepped aboard a Jet Ski and set a course for a ship that was about to turn a million fish into medicine. The throttle on my craft was tetchy and tuned for the fine-motor skills of a younger man. Just a bit of juice and *varoom!* I shot over a wave crest and landed *boom!* in a trough. A zap of pain shot through my lower back and on up into my shoulders. I barely managed to regain my balance before another wave broke across the bow and threatened to dump me into the Chesapeake Bay.

Blazing out ahead was my guide, a man a few years older than I but perfectly in tune with his machine. Brian Lockwood was known in the fishing towns of coastal Virginia as Jet Ski Brian. My trip with him was to be one of a dozen sorties he'd make in the days ahead. *Blam blam blam* he'd go over the wave crests, all week long. He was absolutely loving his job. Actually, he didn't even really consider it a job. Technically, Brian had finished with real work, having mysteriously created and sold something for a retirement-size amount of money.

At a certain point, Jet Ski Brian realized his client had fallen too far behind. He waved, circled back, and rubbed his hand through his thick salt-and-pepper hair.

"Takes a little getting used to," he said, and then made a surprisingly squeaky little laugh, like a mouse.

"Yeah," I managed through gritted teeth. "How much farther?"

"We-ell let's take a look-see," he said, just the slightest bit of the South in his mid-Atlantic accent. He fingered the cracked iPhone mounted to his transom and zoomed in on a pair of red dots. "I'm seeing one Omega boat pretty close over here, and another one up off the shoal over there. I'm not sure how long this one here is going to be on the menhaden, but we should run into him in an hour or so."

An hour or so? I thought.

But what I said was, "Cool."

Off again we tore across the waves, and eventually I dared to hold the throttle steady regardless of the next wave's impact. What the hell? Brian had driven one of these things all the way to the Bahamas. Why was he weathering middle age so much better than I? And where was his great enthusiasm coming from? We were objectively similar people. We both had organized our lives around the sea. I'd written two whole books about fish, for Christ's sake. Yet while Brian seemed to be drawing more and more energy from the miraculous ocean, I felt as if I were slipping beneath its surface.

These kinds of ruminations were what had led me to Jet Ski Brian in the first place. I had sought him out because he promised he could help me witness the extraction of a substance that had lately come to occupy my thoughts—a substance upon which I had unwittingly built an entire career. This substance, this host of molecules, hadn't much concerned me when I was younger. In fact, I often bridled when my older readership mentioned it. They were fixated on it, obsessed, to the exclusion of all other matters relating to the sea. But now as I rounded the corner of my forty-seventh birthday and caught sight of fifty in the middle distance, that substance had started to come more clearly into focus.

It had all begun as a whisper, speaking to me most clearly late at night—a quiet murmur of dread over the nature of middle age and what lay beyond it. It felt as if an entirely new phase had begun, something which I had come to think of as "the rind of life"—a phase of insomnia and pointless internet browsing leading to dark speculation on the paucity of time remaining and the declining vitality that would accompany this last handful of decades. Late one evening, a search of one of my fish books led me to click on the geographical distribution of that book's sales. There was an unnatural rise in the state of Utah. Why were so many people buying fish books in the mountains? A deep Google dive revealed a listing for a trade association in Salt Lake City called GOED: a "Global Organization" for eicosapentaenoic and docosahexaenoic fatty acids, commonly abbreviated as EPA and DHA—the two most famous members of a family of molecules known collectively as the omega-3s.

More insomnia. Shortness of breath. Fast heartbeats. Slow thinking. Searches for homeopathic cures for depression. Dietary ways of addressing anxiety. Supplements that might shift things. Once more links pointed back to GOED.

I had written about omega-3s in an offhand kind of way. When I wanted to make a point that a particular fish was a "good choice," I would often check that fish's omega-3 levels. The ones that had higher numbers I always put on a list of fish to use for what I came to think of as "The Standard Article." The article titled "Smart, Sustainable Choices from the Sea," subtitle: "Our oceans are in trouble, but these five seafoods can help you improve your health and save the planet." Which fish should I eat? Why these, of course. They're sustainable. *And* they are very high in omega-3s.

But what *was* the omega-3? What did it actually do in the human body? Why was it always mentioned but never satisfactorily explained?

More rumination. A search for the phrase "omega-3s may . . ." produced a wide range of speculations. Omega-3s may "help prevent coronary heart disease," "increase brain volume," "boost sperm competitiveness," "build muscle in older adults," "prevent some forms of depression," "help lower risk of type 2 diabetes." Many hypotheses. Many academic papers. Taken collectively, they promised no less than a cure for middle age.

Built within all those many health claims was cause for what some referred to as a global health crisis. For if you were to take all of the fish of the world, boil them down, and produce the necessary pills to supplement the world's anticipated nine billion humans with the amount of eicosapentaenoic and docosahexaenoic omega-3 fatty acids advocates say we'd need to lead healthy lives, the ocean would have to be mercilessly raided. Bold innovation was required. It had to come. Because many in the medical community had concluded that omega-3s were "essential" fatty acids—dietarily essential because humans cannot make them, or not much of them, anyway. We mainly get them into our body by eating them. Many physicians also deemed them essential because they are crucial components of important organs like the brain and eyes. In fact DHA makes up 5 to 10 percent of the human brain's weight. And after nearly thirty thousand medical studies, some health professionals had concluded that the risk of cardiovascular disease could be reduced by anywhere from 9 to 30 percent by taking the golden pill. Surely we would all suffer if we couldn't solve the omega-3 problem.

Or was it a problem?

Until very recently it was hard to find anything that disputed the omega-3-as-essential-nutrient narrative. But in 2012, a number of long-term studies commissioned back in the molecules' popular ascendance reached completion. One by one the studies accumulated. A 2012 meta-analysis by Evangelos C. Rizos and colleagues published in the normally definitive *Journal of the American Medical Association* reviewed nearly two dozen of the recent studies. Its conclusion: omega-3 supplementation "was not associated with a lower risk of all-cause mortality, cardiac death, sudden death, myocardial infarction, or stroke based on relative and absolute measures of association."

But this could not stop the omega-3 juggernaut. The industry continued to grow. As of this writing, omega-3s already ranked among the world's most profitable dietary supplements. Sunnier market analyses predicted sales would increase by a rate of more than 7 percent per year for the foreseeable future. Every year more and more trials were being published, to the point where omega-3s rank with many vitamins as some of the most studied organic molecules on earth.

It went beyond just the supplement industry. The fishing industry and the newly emergent seafood farming industry (known in the marine business community as aquaculture) also hung their hopes on the omega-3s. Aquaculture, the human-guided husbandry of everything from kelp to codfish, has since the 1980s been the fastest-growing food system on the planet, and one of the primary justifications for its growth is the purported need for more omega-3s in the Western diet.

But as I dug deeper, another aspect of the omega-3s emerged that raised significant questions beyond the realm of human health. The ultimate creators of omega-3s—the original build-ers of this set of molecules that so obsesses us today—are not fish, but phytoplankton, the creatures that underlie the entire oceanic food web. So significant are these microorganisms that they function as a shadow weather system. They create half of the world's breathable oxygen, and an equally impressive amount of the world's carbon at one time or another passes through their membranes. A single species of phytoplankton, called *Prochlorococcus,* is the most abundant living thing on earth. It contains four times as many genes as human DNA—genes that could address numerous ecological problems if hu-mans could only figure out a way to properly manipulate them. *Prochlorococcus* is one of the primary ways solar energy enters the ocean food web and gets transferred to higher life. Thirty years ago, we didn't even know *Prochlorococcus* existed.

But as go phytoplankton, so goes the world. A recent peer-reviewed study estimated that the 2.5-degree increase in ocean temperatures we are likely to see in the next half century will reduce planktonic sources of omega-3s by as much as 25 percent. As a middle-aged man, I was troubled by the idea of a Big One striking me down. In a sense, though, the ocean is reaching its own midlife, approaching its four billionth birthday in a life that will likely span nine billion years. What if the sea was on course for a midlife Big One of its own?

As I put all this together, the contours of an exploration started to take shape. What if I was to journey to the corners of the world where most of the omega-3 harvesting and research occurred? Darkest Peru. Farthest Antarctica. The tippy top of Norway. Even right next door along my home coast of Connecticut, where some of the earliest studies of omega-3s and plankton had taken place. There I would get to know the creatures most people had never heard of but that were the backbone of a multibillion-dollar industry. Chesapeake Bay menhaden, Peruvian anchoveta, Antarctic krill—these were the ignominious things that were scooped up whole schools at a time, the raw material of a global industry that together with the animal feed and fertilizer industries removed from the base of the marine food web nearly the equivalent of the human weight of the United States each and every year. Regulators and corporate executives that oversaw all of this harvesting continue to insist that much of this extraction is sustainable. But what would the world look like, I wondered, if an extra fifty-four billion pounds of life were kept in the oceans instead of being boiled down into fertilizer, animal feed, and dietary supplements?

Beyond fishing, I knew I might well observe larger

environmental changes on an omega journey. If I were to em-
bark on such an exploration could I not get a glimpse of how
profoundly things were changing—how the sea was warming,
how its cycles were shifting and its chemistry coming apart? If
I looked long and hard at the very bottom of marine food webs
in all these places, at all these humble fish and crustaceans and
plankton, rich in their long-chain fatty acids, perhaps I would
gain a perspective on the sea that I lacked. Perhaps the omega-3
was a path to a better understanding of the ocean.

The more I examined the question of the omega-3, the
more I realized that there was a story here that circled back to
human health *and* the health of the planet—something that
was immediately apparent when I drove down to the Chesapeake Bay to meet up with Jet Ski Brian. Thick in the air was
the smell of chicken and pig manure, the factory farms pushing
relentlessly down to the bay. All along the lowlands were rows
and rows of corn and soy, commodity crops that fed all those
animals. Today, in spite of the fact that fish is widely touted for
its health benefits, Americans manage to eat only around 15
pounds of it per year, compared with 210 pounds of land food
meat. This doesn't take into account the overwhelming tonnage of corn, soy, wheat, rice, and other land-based plants that
are the bulk of the American diet. Once, we existed on food
that was essentially in tune with the ocean and the omega-
3-based chemistry that grew out of its depths. In the last century, though, we have retooled both the chemistry and the
biology of the planet to accommodate what we now think of as
the "Western diet"—a diet that in turn is criticized by nutritionists for its correlation with a range of chronic diseases.

What would it mean for both planetary health and human health if instead of working *against* the energy of the sea, we worked *with* it? What would happen if we followed a kind of omega principle where we figured out a way to make the omega-3 not just a supplement that we took to balance out our other bad behaviors but rather the basis for a new human diet? What would an omega-3 world look like? More urgent for the person hitting middle age, what would human health look like in a world where omega-3s were the core of the food system rather than relegated to a corner of a supplement shop?

In my heart of hearts—as well as for the sake of my actual beating heart—I did indeed want what "The Standard Article" promised. I *did* want a way of eating that saved me but also saved the sea. Opinions about the causes of modern chronic illness vary, but there is one overall opinion that dietitians, epidemiologists, family physicians, agronomists, and marine ecologists generally share: the way we eat in the West is out of balance. In deciding to follow the omega-3 from its emergence on the planet to the dietary and environmental predicaments of our present era, I had a hunch and a hope that the path toward balance would reveal itself.

Which was why I found myself skimming across the surface of the Chesapeake Bay that hot July morning. Throttling down behind Jet Ski Brian, I saw a big blue ship owned by Omega Protein, the largest reducer of menhaden in the United States. The vessel was a creation of the industrial age called a purse seiner, named for the particular way it surrounds a school of fish and pockets the sea's treasure. Above me a spotter plane circled in the clear sky, the sun glinting off its wings, its pilot radioing down the coordinates of the menhaden school to the skipper below. Soon small aluminum boats were lowered from the mother vessel into the water. A blow of a horn. An encircling of the school of thousands of little lives with the purse seine. A second horn. The drawing tight of the purse. The air thick with the odd watermelon smell of fresh menhaden, the fish panicking into a froth as the net drew tight around them. A loading of those lives onto an aluminum ladder that brought them aboard the main vessel. The cascade of those lives, a silver waterfall, into a dark hold below.

All of it to be boiled down into an oil that some believed would help us be much better than we are.

One

ALGAE'S TOOLS

Whenever I step aboard the Metro-North train from my present home in Manhattan toward my childhood home in coastal Connecticut, I feel as if I am being borne back in time. Past New Rochelle, where my father took me to plumb the bays and inlets for flounder on divorced-dad weekends, through exclusive and excluding Greenwich where I guided a battered little skiff in search of mackerel and bluefish, oblivious in my youth to all the many forces building against the sea. Back then I was happy to be just another predator hunting fish.

But a little while ago the Metro-North out of Grand Central took me much deeper into the past, to a laboratory that has for the last eighty years been investigating some of the world's oldest organisms—organisms that paved the way for my memories and your existence. Indeed, nothing in our world would be as it is today but for these several thousand species of microscopic algae also known as phytoplankton. Not only did they lay the foundation for complexity in the early eons of life on earth, but they also continue to govern the modern cycles of oxygen and carbon that influence our planet's climate. Most relevant to the present account, they are also the creatures that first synthesized the omega-3 fatty acids.

This fact was brought to my attention soon after I detrained at Milford, Connecticut. There I met a man who had spent his life staring into a microscope at the swirling brown and green world that lies at the bottom of everything.

Gary Wikfors is the bemused, white-haired sage who now runs the National Oceanic and Atmospheric Administration's (NOAA) laboratory in Milford. Still filled with a boyish curiosity about the natural world and more than a little bit startled to find himself sixty-two years old, he nevertheless thinks often about the distant past. He is fond of antique musical instruments and can coax a tune out of a good many of them. Like any good scientist, he is hesitant to speculate about something he did not directly observe, but when I asked him about the very beginning of the omega-3 story, he grudgingly complied.

"Well, believe it or not, I wasn't there," he joked. "But phytoplankton are the main organisms on earth that assemble omega-3s de novo. They have the enzymes and the cell machinery to make these fatty acids." The process of creating omega-3s was put in motion, Wikfors explained, by the way early life changed the world.

It begins, as the Hebrew Bible correctly records, with light. Or rather with the way light played upon the sea and how the sea reacted to it. Around 3 billion years ago, a microorganism invented a process that could convert solar energy into chemical bonds: oxygen-producing photosynthesis.

Eventually the descendents of these early photosynthetic organisms came to make a fatty acid called alpha-linolenic acid, or ALA. A short-chain fatty acid, ALA shows up most commonly in the thylakoid membranes of organelles known as chloroplasts. When ALA arrived on the scene earth was cloaked by an insulating blanket of carbon dioxide. As those early photosynthesizers broke CO_2 into its constituent elements, they stripped that blanket away. The atmosphere got both cooler and more oxygenated, bringing about a problem that was in part solved by transforming ALA into what are known as long-chain omega-3 fatty acids.

Omega-3s are unsaturated fats—that is, fats with dynamic, ever-pivoting double bonds between carbon atoms at the ends of their structures. The name "omega" comes from the fact that the first frenetic and freewheeling double bond appears at the omega end of the molecule, three carbons in from the terminus of the fatty acid chain. Their christener, the chemist Ralph Holman, was led to the name in the 1960s from a line in Revelation: "I am the Alpha and the Omega, the first and the last, the beginning and the end," said God to John. Holman liked the powerful biblical resonance, but he also liked the name because, as he told the writer Susan Allport in her excellent history *The Queen of Fats*, "something about *omega* rolls off the tongue easily."

If the word "omega" rolls off the tongue, then the omega-3 fatty acids are similarly fluid. "A membrane's degree of flexibility is largely dependent on what kinds of fats they contain," Gary Wikfors explained. "If the membrane contains high amounts of what are called saturated fatty acids [fat molecules with brittle single carbon bonds], the membrane is stiff. If they are rich in unsaturated fats, like omega-3s, they are fluid."

Why is this important? Like everything in chemistry and in daily experience, things are stiffer when they're cold. At cold temperatures, unsaturated fatty acids make a membrane more flexible. It turns out that as a direct result of the cooler climate—something that early phytoplankton themselves brought about by stripping away all that insulating CO_2—phytoplankton had to change to survive. The omega-3 was a key adaptation that allowed them to keep up with cooler times.

"The expansion of life toward the poles would have been dependent on the ability to maintain membrane fluidity at colder temperatures," Wikfors continued. "Contaminating the poles with life would require that capability."

And contaminate them they did. Phytoplankton radiated far and wide. So numerous were they that we still experience the echo of their abundance every day of our modern lives. The trillions upon trillions of ancient phytoplankton in their fossilized form are literally what drive us: petroleum. Most of the gasoline we burn today began as clumps of plankton.

Indeed, if one was fond of biological conspiracy theories, one could make the case that our present geological age is only very myopically termed the Anthropocene—literally "the age of man." Rather we are at one end of an epic microbial loop. As we burn the billions of gallons of phytoplankton corpses that are now releasing billions of tons of carbon into the atmosphere, we are in effect re-creating the ancient conditions that preceded us. The Anthropocene turns out to be perfect weather for the very earliest microorganisms. Creatures that vastly prefer a hot, carbon-soaked planet.

To show me the importance of the juncture at which omega-3s first arrived on the scene, Wikfors led me into the heart of the NOAA lab, the place where his predecessors had meticulously cataloged phytoplankton species according to their particular characteristics. There in neat rows were two racks of beakers. The top row's beakers had fluids colored shades of murky yellow-brown; the bottom's had liquids of a bright green pigment. These two bottles, it turned out, contained worlds.

"There are two main lines of evolution in phytoplankton, chromophytes and chlorophytes," Wikfors explained. Chromophytes, the ones in the brown bottle, are organisms that use omega-3s in their membranes and store energy as fats. Chlorophytes, meanwhile, use something called omega-6 fatty acids instead. Omega-6s are similar to omega-3s, with the exception that they put their first double carbon bond at the six position in their hydrocarbon chains. This makes the molecule a lot less bendy. Plants that rely more upon omega-6s built stiffer structures that could stand up to the force of gravity outside the ocean. They also figured out how to store energy as sugar and starch in seeds—the main energy source for modern human food. A stiff cell membrane and an ability to make hard, durable seeds were necessary for plants to move from the sea onto land. As we'll see later, this omega-3/omega-6 split marked an important division between seafood and land food—something that strongly affects the nature of human nutrition today.

There was still another evolutionary divergence that

occurred in part because of the omega-3: the division of marine creatures into predators and prey. Early single-celled plankton called dinoflagellates were probably a key driver of this divergence. Dinoflagellates often contain organelles called plastids. In some dinoflagellates, plastids perform photosynthesis. But in others their light-gathering equipment was retooled to *react* to light rather than simply to absorb it. In these cases, the plastids came to form a kind of early eye that had the ability to sense how light is refracted as it moves through translucent prey. This adaptation helped the dinoflagellates hunt down their food. And, yes, the early dinoflagellate eye was probably high in DHA omega-3 fatty acid.

Today, the predator/prey split in the plankton community is key for stable ocean ecosystems. In modern marine environments, photosynthetic phytoplankton are light-triggered and begin to bloom when the sun's rays first start to lengthen. Soon after, when the water warms, predatory zooplankton bloom. And soon after that, larval fish hatch and consume zooplankton. In this way, solar energy is redirected upward to ever more complex forms of life. If this relationship was ever to be disrupted, it would mean the collapse of fisheries everywhere.

Further up the food chain, the ability of omega-3s to facilitate energy transfer across cell membranes probably aided the spread of fish around the globe. Omega-3s tend to be concentrated in the red muscle tissue fish use for hard, continuous swimming. It is in part for this reason that the fish highest in omega-3s—herring, anchovies, and other members of the order of fish called Clupeiformes—tend to be migratory, schooling animals that are constantly on the move. In such fish, where rapid-fire use of nerve tissue is needed for long hauls, the omega-3 appears to have an important role. Even during periods of poor food availability, fish will hold on to the omega-3s they eat rather than digest them. Other fats get chopped down into simple two-carbon units when eaten, the energy contained within those bonds burned in respiration. Not so for omega-3s. Somewhere, somehow in the course of evolution, nature figured out a way to have fish bodies say, "Wait. Hold on just a sec. Don't burn those. *Those* we can use."

The truth is that most animals, land and sea, need omega-3s but can't really make much of them. This, Gary Wikfors told me, is due to the fact that phytoplankton were so good at synthesizing them and so incredibly numerous that the entire animal kingdom was happy to outsource the process. And so most animals developed what Wikfors calls a selective retention of unsaturated fatty acids, a strategy of conserving rather than creating omega-3s.

The marine biology team at the Milford Lab realized this way back in the 1930s, when they started to decode the phytoplanktonic world. Species by species, culture by culture, the team built one of the world's first "libraries" of microalgae. This was one of the earliest steps in humanity's ongoing project to tame the ocean—a transformation that could have major repercussions for our diet and the balance of life on the planet.

Intimate to understanding how to grow seafood in captivity was a realization of how critical omega-3s were to the growth of nerve cells, for it is in the membranes of nerve cells that omega-3s may play their most crucial role. The principal omega-3 in brain structure is what is called a phospholipid, where strong positive and negative sides of the molecule compel a certain kind of alignment. As Susan Allport explains in *The Queen of Fats*, DHA forms cell membranes that are in effect "lipid sandwiches" in which "the negative phosphate groups (the bread) . . . group themselves on the outside . . . and the fatty tails (the peanut butter) . . . bury themselves in the middle." The more DHA present, the more porous the membrane. Because DHA has six very active double carbon bonds, an added flexibility is granted to the membrane, "providing room for enzymes to maneuver and proteins to twist and turn." This finding led the chemist A. J. Hulbert to conclude that the presence of DHA in human cells "will likely speed up in a relatively nonspecific manner many processes catalyzed by membrane proteins." In other words, the bendy, dynamic DHA omega-3 acid that originally came about to make algae membranes flexible enough to survive a colder planet developed a second purpose much later on in evolutionary history: in complex, multicellular organisms with advanced nervous systems DHA was used to build faster brains.

This is why DHA is particularly abundant in brain cells, where it facilitates not only cognition, but also perception of light. In addition to being an important part of membrane structure, DHA helps in the formation of what are called ion channels in cell signaling—the circuitry underlying an animal's neural network. The early eye in those ancient dinoflagellates I mentioned a few paragraphs back set the course for ever more complex ways of directing chemical messages from cell to cell. It is therefore no surprise that DHA omega-3s are a critical structural element in the photoreceptors of the modern eye. In fact the very early appearance of light-sensitive cells in ancient organisms suggests that the brain may have actually grown in concert with the eye.

It is with the evolution of higher brains, particularly human brains, that the debates around omega-3s start to get prickly. That the eye, and the brain that grew out of it, are deeply dependent on DHA omega-3s is not disputed. But if we follow that argument to its logical conclusion it seems to imply that increasing omega-3s in the diet could increase the speed of cognition. This contentious conclusion hinges on a radical question: could it be that an infusion of seafood deep in prehistory propelled humankind forward to become the savvy, dominating animals we are today?

The first omega-3 studies of the brain began with a physician named Michael Crawford. In the 1960s Crawford journeyed to Kampala, Uganda, to study dietary deficiencies in African tribes that led to rickets and other maladies. In the course of his research, he started looking at the wide array of mammals in Africa and the differences in their brain sizes.

Upon returning to England, he began a detailed analysis of forty-four different mammalian brains and found that no matter what the species, DHA comprised the same proportion of the brain's overall volume. He concluded that the amount of DHA a creature consumed was in lockstep with the size of an animal's brain and went so far as to propose that humans must have evolved their big brains shoreside, where ample supplies of shellfish could be obtained with minimal expenditure of energy.

When I imagine this hypothesis at work, I see a raw and

blustery afternoon tens of thousands of years in the past. A small group of humans is huddled in the recess of a sea cliff as the last of a series of winter storms blows a gray ceiling of clouds out over the Indian Ocean. Genetically it has been estimated that the human race dwindled to isolated pockets that could have numbered as few as two thousand individuals somewhere in the period from 70,000–35,000 BCE. In such a scenario it is easy to picture a tiny, overwhelmed clutch of lost souls awaiting their demise. They would already have had the beginnings of complex thought, but the neurons that fired within those big brains might have led to unimaginative conclusions. They would have had some social skills, had the ability and the proclivity to associate, but quarrels, anger, and the darkest of depressions kept them at each other's throats. The dawn of humanity was not so far in the past, but had these few remaining humans not radically changed their ways, the species' dusk would have come in a matter of months.

What might have occurred at this crucial moment was that one individual felt the sea in her nose and was drawn to the cove that lay just beyond the cave. Wading into the water, she inched her way along the rocks with her toughened feet and calloused hands, only to find a few of the rocks slightly loose. She felt the slightest bit of elation when one easily pulled away—like a fruit or a berry plucked from a bush. She shook it against her ear and sensed something sloshing inside. Holding it up to her nose, she smelled the vaguest hint of meat. She gathered more. When she returned to the encampment, she threw the booty she'd taken from the sea into the last embers of a dying fire. The flames sputtered at first, in danger of going out. Suddenly, a hiss and a pop came from the stones. Miraculously they opened, revealing mollusk meat within. Falling on the morsels of warm food, the humans devoured it all. When they had pulled every last mussel from its shell, they made foray after foray to the water's edge and ate still more. After the feast had been consumed, for the first time in many months they were sated and, perhaps, even a little bit happy.

A vignette like this would be something you would imagine if you subscribed to what has come to be called the aquatic ape hypothesis. Michael Crawford did not propose it, but his work on omega-3s and brains forms one of the hypothesis's cornerstones. Its adherents have even suggested that the human ability to walk on two feet was linked to a semiaquatic lifestyle. Early hominids, the argument goes, would never have learned to stand up to gravity had they not felt the lightening effect of wading out into water to gather shellfish.

Contrarians abound, of course. Observers of aboriginal peoples today raise the question: if omega-3s are so important to the brain, why are there perfectly intelligent tribal societies living hundreds of miles from the sea who have never had a bite of seafood? In one analysis in the *British Journal of Nutrition*, the clinician John Langdon argued that both nursing mothers and their infants "have mechanisms to store and buffer the supply of DHA" on their own without any seafood in their diet and concluded that "the hypothesis that DHA has been a limiting resource in human brain evolution must be considered to be unsupported."

To this contrary view there are some answers, chiefly lying in a series of chemical reactions that have been gradually decoded over the last fifty years. While land plants do not contain long-chain EPA and DHA fatty acids, some do contain in their leaves small amounts of alpha-linolenic acid—the very same ALA that forms precursors to long-chain omega-3s in ocean-based plants. It turns out that animals, including humans, can in the right dietary context upgrade ALA into long-chain EPA and then DHA. Conceivably, a Paleolithic population that had at the center of its diet large amounts of wild ALA-rich field greens could metabolize enough DHA to think.

Whatever the means to achieving high levels of DHA in our brains, something changed in human thinking in relatively recent history. Yuval Harari posits in his book *Sapiens* that somewhere between 70,000 and 30,000 years ago BCE a "cognitive revolution" took place that led to a marked expansion of our ability to imagine and create. And there is some evidence suggesting that seafood could have been part of that revolution. In 2007 the remnants of sixty-thousand-year-old seafood feasts were discovered in a cave at Pinnacle Point, South Africa. In those same caves, archaeologists noted the presence of paintings far more complex than cave art from similar periods. Researchers hypothesized from these findings that the tiny tribe that occupied the point could have achieved greater social stability and higher levels of development in part because they made seafood central to their diet.

Another broader argument for the link between seafood intake and higher cognition is an odd coincidence that occurred more recently throughout humankind's geographical range. Our species came to eat significant amounts of ocean protein much later than land food game. Our turn to the ocean seems to have coincided with the moment when we overhunted large land mammals to the point where they could no longer support our dietary needs. A notable intensification of marine foraging is marked in the archaeological record by huge shell piles and fishbone middens dated to around 8000 BCE, just about the same time that land food game started to dwindle and sea levels began to fall. And shortly after that, the first signs of agriculture began to appear.

Where is the causation and where is the correlation here? Did humans turn to seafood as a last-ditch hunting strategy before going full bore into agriculture? Or did seafood and the omega-3s it provided give us a cognitive leg up that moved us toward more technologically complex ways of obtaining food? We can't know for sure, of course. What we do know is that agriculture first appeared in six centers around the world between 10,000 and 5,000 BCE: Mesopotamia, coastal New Guinea, coastal China, coastal Peru, coastal Mexico, and along the Mississippi River. These centers appear to have arisen independently of one another, but they all share one attribute: proximity to fish and shellfish. And, curiously, these centers were accompanied by a second innovation that rests upon an uptick in cognition: the precursors to modern language. The major language groups of the world correspond more or less to the six different agricultural centers. The archaeological record reveals very little innovation during humanity's first 200,000 years on earth. And then all of a sudden, boom: agriculture, advanced communication, structurally complex society.

Whether seafood was at the root of this leap, the species

changed and a DHA-rich brain was a part of that change. Terrestrial agriculture spread rapidly. Early farmers isolated and
cultivated the descendants of those first chlorophyte plants.
They launched a haphazard breeding program, selecting vari-
eties for their ability to make starch and omega-6-rich seeds.
The wild, grass-browsing game they hunted became less and
less central to their diet. The early forms of today's commodity
crops—corn, soy, wheat, and rice—arose as the central pillars
of human nutrition. This dramatic infusion of high-energy
carbohydrates didn't necessarily make those first farmers live
longer, healthier lives than their hunter-gatherer antecedents.
Rather it gave a boost of strength to the young among them,
allowing them to raise larger families, who in turn became
farmers and spread this new high-carbohydrate diet around
the globe.

But there was one place in the world where grass-browsing
mammals and wild fish continued to be intermingled significantly with farmed grains. That place was also among the first
regions where philosophy and advanced civilization took hold,
indeed where medicine itself was born: the Mediterranean.

Two

THE SEA BETWEEN
THE LANDS

The Mediterranean presents itself as a perfect expression of balance. Ideally poised between alpine coolness to the north and the blazing Sahara to the south, it is that special sweet spot that allowed humanity to blossom. In September it seems particularly well calibrated, and the rind of life feels sweet and mellow and stripped entirely of its bitterness. Hours drift by in a succession of sharp-edged days and temperate nights. The sea is at its briniest, and swimming upon the gentle waves one feels positively buoyed by the crystal-clear blueness, enjoying views of the surrounding cliffs and the traces of the Roman aqueducts that still snake their way from high mountain meadows. The cafés are empty, restaurant staffs are pleasant, and there is ample time to pick apart a complicated issue over a long meal.

On just such a September morning I'd been slowly making my way toward the Italian fishing village of Cetara, a town built into a rocky crevice twenty-five miles southeast of Naples.

I was headed there because I wanted to more fully understand the essence of Mediterranean balance. Cetara's province of Salerno is legendary for its residents' longevity. In one of its villages, Acciaroli, 10 percent of the inhabitants are over a hundred years old. A third of those hundred-year-olds are past 110. A possible cause of all of those spry hundred-plusers? A product in which the town of Cetara takes particular pride: the European anchovy, *Engraulis encrasicolus,* a small member of the order Clupeiformes whose annual migrations up and down the Amalfi Coast make it a bedrock of the local cuisine. Like so many Italian towns, Cetara has decided to stake its reputation, even its very soul, on a single food product. Just as the region around Parma has its cheese and Perugia its chocolate, so Cetara has its anchovy. In the spirit of a local food movement that is much more intense than any in America, Cetarans have zeroed in on this silvery minnowlike fish—a fish with exceptionally high levels of omega-3 fatty acids.

After I had waited for an hour at a station in Salerno, the bus to Cetara finally alighted, and a crush of young Italian bodies spread-eagled me against the interior wall. Soon we began the long slow climb toward Amalfi. Four shirtless college-age boys, their shoulders and chests taut with young muscle, claimed the whole back bench, rotated their baseball caps to a perfect angle, and started playing an Italian rap song on their iPhone speakers. Without a care they rapped along, twirling their hands in syncopated rhythm while equally young and beautiful women decried the song choice. Three-quarters of the way up one hill, the bus stopped and opened its doors. A man about my age took a moment's pause when he saw the density of the youth before him. Then he dipped his shoulder and rammed himself inside.

A dozen "*ma noooooooooos*" erupted from the young Italians in protest.

"*Eh ragazzi,*" the middle-aged man shouted back angrily. "*E cosi!*"

I couldn't agree with you more, brother, I thought. "It is what it is."

Through switchback after switchback the bus rattled on before finally grinding its overtaxed gears to a stop at Cetara, where I was belched onto the sidewalk. I had been instructed to find a restaurant called Acquapazza—Crazy Water—and as if on command, a white van depicting a naked classical hero with a giant penis ending in the shape of an anchovy blew past. ACQUAPAZZA, the van's logo declared. I followed the anchovy penis van up a hill and there spied Beatrice Ughi, the woman who had promised to unlock the secrets of the Cetara anchovy for me and help me understand how the fish fit more broadly into what has come to be called the Mediterranean Diet.

"Paul," Beatrice had written me before I'd left for Italy, "I have just been speaking with our friends at Nettuno. They tell me that we can come on the fourteenth and fifteenth of September to visit Cetara. There you will see the production happening. And *then*, after meeting with the mayor, Mayor Secondo Squizzatto (what a name!), and with the head of the anchovy association, Pietro Pesce (perfect, no?), we will discuss the situation with the anchovies of Cetara and, if the conditions are right, maybe, *may*be we will fish the anchovies. I myself really need to go. I really need to see the process and to make sure that they are doing it exactly right as they promise they are doing."

This attention to detail was in keeping with Beatrice's mid-life re-creation of herself. She had emigrated to the United States in the late 1980s, transferring from the Rome office to the New York office of her corporate accounting firm. She'd happily married an older American businessman and, like many other women at the time, had subsisted entirely on a diet of SlimFast. "I knew the food was going to be terrible in New York," she'd told me. "And so I didn't really care what I ate." But as she approached fifty, she changed direction on a whim. It was the time of the rise of Carlo Petrini and his Slow Food movement, a time when food was suddenly reborn. To eat well was to be well. This idea captivated Beatrice as she considered what to do with her own life's rind.

With the acumen and tightfistedness of a lifelong accountant, Beatrice established a small business in an outpost in the South Bronx and slowly built what is arguably the best Italian specialty food importer in the United States, an institution called Gustiamo. In short, Beatrice does pretty much exactly what any member of Western civilization seeking a second career in midlife would hope to do: she travels to Italy several times a year, rigorously interrogates the integrity of her producers, and returns home to New York with the most delicious natural food the Mediterranean has to offer.

It was Beatrice who had insisted that Cetara was the place for me to understand the Mediterranean and its role in the omega-3 story. As she and her colleague Danielle sat down with me at Ristorante Acquapazza, I felt I had made the right choice. Soon we were joined by the restaurant's founders: two cousins, each called Gennaro. One Gennaro was wide chested and expansive in his gestures. The other Gennaro was lean and spare and, despite having just turned fifty, sported a thick thatch of floppy blond hair, cut *Rubber Soul*–era Beatles style. Before long, dishes began appearing, each different in its use of anchovies. Freshly grilled anchovies practically bursting with their own oil. Cured anchovies with sharply salty olives. Broccoli cooked in an anchovy-based sauce spritzed with a grassy-scented spray of fresh olive oil.

As we finished our meal and espresso came, Beatrice took the helm of the conversation and turned it to what she knew was on my mind.

"So tell me, Gennaro, what do you think? What is your opinion of this *omega tre*?"

"*Omega tre*?"

"Omega-3!" Beatrice said in English and gestured to the village at large. "Yes, do you take this pill?"

"I've heard of it. This omega-3. But no, I would never take it."

"Ha-ha. Why not?"

Here he looked around the escarpments and quays as if asking the countryside itself to give a reply. "Look," he said, "I live in a little village of twenty-five hundred souls. And I know it seems like we are a provincial sort of place. But some of the things that I hear, in particular those things that come from evolved countries like America, surprise me. We are very influenced by trends that come from America. But when it comes to food, I think we are, I'm sorry, a bit more advanced. You, you are from America, yes?"

"Yes," I admitted.

"This is what you do there: you take something that is completely normal and good. But instead of just leaving it as it is you try to make a business out of it. You take it and make it into a trend."

"*Ma aspetta*"—wait—Gennaro Number Two interjected. "It's science, too. They are collaborating over at the University of Naples with some of our products. They *are* looking at the omega-3."

"Sure, maybe they are, but I tell you this," Gennaro Number One said. "It's very simple. When I go to Tuscany and eat meat for three days and I don't eat fish, I feel weird. They shouldn't study the omega-3, they should study the *people* and how we *feel*."

In fact, what Gennaro Number One was proposing has been the subject of intense scientific inquiry for the last sixty years throughout the Mediterranean: the essential fissure running through the diets of modern societies and their ancient forebears.

The first of these inquiries began just after World War II on the island of Crete. It didn't begin as an attempt to try to understand how well Mediterranean people ate. Rather, American investigators were invited to Crete by the Greek government to try to "improve" the diets of Greeks. The Greek islanders had suffered a long slog of guerrilla fighting during World War II and an equally difficult and bitter civil war.

During the chaos they had reverted to a subsistence diet that was probably quite close to the original foods early Mediterranean people ate. Greek officials were concerned that Cretans were dangerously malnourished. Led by the epidemiologist Leland Allbaugh and funded by the Rockefeller Foundation, investigators fanned out across the land of old King Minos and set about inventorying the food of one out of every 150 households.

The researchers found that the food system of Crete was a sparing one. Unlike the industrial-scale farms of the American Great Plains, the Mediterranean island plots were small and had never had sophisticated forms of fertilization and irrigation. Their overall output was meager, comparable in caloric output to early hunter-gatherer slash-and-burn attempts at agriculture.

Cretans were hardly enjoying this Spartan regime. "We are hungry most of the time," one subject told Allbaugh. Most of the survey respondents listed meat as their favorite food even though they rarely ate it. What Cretans were actually eating was another story. The modest protein component of the diet came from wild fish or pasture-raised animals that browsed on wild field greens. The diet's fat came from olive trees that preserved much of the land in a semiforested state that in turn held the soil together and conserved moisture. Carbohydrates came from whole grains grown on small-parcel farms that produced adequate but not overwhelming amounts of starch. Legumes, too, supplemented the diet, but they were there as much to help other crops fix nitrogen in the poor soil as they were to supply nutrition. There was also an unusually high amount of leafy greens in the diet, especially in more mountainous areas where soils were particularly poor. In spite of the persistent feeling of hunger, adherents to this diet lived longer and had markedly lower incidences of cardiovascular diseases than their American counterparts. Over time, clinicians began circling a concept that embodied the Cretan way of eating.

Leading the way in synthesizing and extending the lessons of Crete was a quixotic researcher named Ancel Keys. Keys came to the Mediterranean in a roundabout way. He was a polymath of the highest order. He had been labeled a genius at thirteen years of age and made part of a longitudinal genius study that would continue for eighty-five years of his life. In a long career that wended its way through the military (he would invent the soldier's chow called the K-ration), the Himalayas (he would do a long-term study on the effect of altitude), and hunger (he would lead an infamous study at the University of Minnesota that forcibly starved conscientious objectors), he would eventually end up on Italian shores near Salerno. There, he and his wife, Margaret, started to zero in on what would prove to be his most enduring legacy.

Keys first became interested in the Mediterranean style of eating when an Italian delegate at a Food and Agriculture Organization of the United Nations conference on hunger in Rome reported that there was barely any incidence of heart disease in Naples and the surrounding towns. This stayed on Keys's mind throughout a dreary series of winters, and finally, while on sabbatical teaching at Oxford, he and his wife decided they needed a change. Abandoning England for a drive down the Italian coast, they did something they had not expected to do at their age. They fell in love.

As he crossed over to Italy from Switzerland, Keys noted that on the Italian side of the Alps, "the air was mild, flowers were gay, birds were singing. . . . We felt warm all over." He was struck by the amount of fresh vegetables and fruit in Italian meals and only a "modest portion of meat or fish perhaps twice a week." That and olive oil. Always olive oil, served raw, or cooked, or over salads and seafood.

Keys would go on to conduct research in Italy where he compared the blood, diets, and lifestyles of laborers with low incidence of heart attacks to those of white-collar executives with higher incidence and found that serum cholesterol (in the blood) was higher for executives than laborers. This discovery eventually led to the much-cited Seven Countries Study based on the hypothesis that diet, particularly consumption of saturated fat, was related to adult men's risk of coronary heart disease. As an initial result, the so-called Mediterranean Diet, with a high intake of monounsaturated olive oil and little consumption of saturated fats, was credited with being the best for a low incidence of coronary heart disease. Keys and his biochemist wife published three books based on his research, including the two bestsellers: *Eat Well and Stay Well* (1959) and *How to Eat Well and Stay Well the Mediterranean Way* (1975).

Keys and his insistence on the evils of saturated fats captured the public's dietary attention at the time, leading discussions around coronary heart disease to focus on what was perceived essentially as a plumbing problem. Saturated fats get their name from the fact that hydrogen atoms attach to all the available carbon bonds in the fat molecule, thus "saturating" it and causing it to have a much higher melting point than unsaturated fats. This solid, unmelting lipid material was thus thought to be literally plugging up the works. Olive oil, Keys thought, was the fluid solution.

That olive oil played a role in the Mediterranean Diet's positive effects seems to be true. But there are some clinicians who believe it is the balance of *all* the fats in the human diet that ultimately governs cardiovascular health and that the ideal fat balance was achieved in the Mediterranean by following a regime that was similar, at least in terms of lipid intake, to the diet of the region's early hunter-gatherers. This position is perhaps most ardently taken by a Greek cardiologist named appropriately after the Hellenic goddess of the hunt.

Artemis Simopoulos grew up in the shadow of Ancel Keys and his theories about fats. But she took issue with his way of thinking, mostly because it didn't address the ways the human body actually processed fat and the way fat acted as a dynamic chemical compound rather than a physical stopper in the plumbing of the human body. "I met Ancel Keys," Simopoulos told me over a murky dark cup of Greek coffee emblazoned with an illustration of the Parthenon. "Keys wasn't a physician. He didn't understand human metabolism. All Keys cared about was saturated fat. And in the end *he* was fat."

The overbearing presence of Keys and his cholesterol obsession bothered Simopoulos so much that she began an analysis of the Greek version of the Mediterranean Diet. While teaching at the Mediterranean Agronomic Institute of Chania, she went back to some of the original Seven Country Study data and made further analyses of what she thought was the true model for eating. She found a marked difference—in particular, the presence of a succulent called purslane.

Purslane is a plant that grows wild throughout the rough terrain of the Greek islands and coastal headlands. Simopoulos noticed it one day in the 1970s when she happened to be staying at her family's country home in the southern Peloponnese. During that visit she started watching the habits of the local chickens that most villagers kept in their yards. Almost to a bird, she noticed, they showed a preference for purslane. How, Simopoulos wondered, would this be reflected in the chemical composition of chickens and eggs? Realizing that U.S. customs would never allow her to smuggle a chicken back into the United States, she gathered up a dozen eggs, hard-boiled them, and put them in her handbag as a "snack" supposedly to be eaten on the plane.

Back in the lipid lab at the National Institutes of Health, she and Dr. Norman Salem set about doing a profile of the Greek eggs. She did the same with eggs that had come from grain-fed, industrially raised American chickens. The difference between the two was intriguing. The Greek egg had a lipid profile similar to what one would find in the egg of a wild bird. It had high amounts of omega-3s and a modest amount of another omega—the omega-6 fatty acid. But when she looked at the American egg she was struck by a profound imbalance. The American egg showed a ratio of omega-6 to omega-3 of twenty-to-one. Soon she realized this imbalance appeared everywhere in the American diet. Notably off-kilter were the cooking oils in which Americans drowned their food. Corn oil: sixty-six-to-one. Soy, the most prevalent oil of all: twelve-to-one. Taken collectively, this unbalancing influx of omega-6-leaning cooking oil amounted to what one clinician at the National Institutes of Health told me was "the largest single change to the American diet in the last hundred years."

Simopoulos believed this was a critical dietary mistake, primarily because an overabundance of omega-6 can lead to inflammation. Inflammation is one of the chief ways the body prepares itself to defend against microbial attack. It begins when capillaries dilate, opening a gateway for white blood cells to launch a counterattack against bacteria and viruses. The problems with inflammation begin when it doesn't subside. Extended periods of inflammation put pressure on nerves and also possibly stimulate pain receptors in affected areas. Inflammation has been implicated in cardiovascular disease, dementia, cancer, type 2 diabetes, and arthritis. The fact that Mediterranean people have generally lower rates of all these diseases implied that somehow the Mediterranean eating pattern addressed inflammation. Indeed, some have taken to calling the Mediterranean Diet an anti-inflammation diet.

And this is where omega-6s come in. Omega-6s include arachidonic acid, which is a precursor for compounds called prostaglandins that in some reactions can be inflammatory. Prior to beginning her own investigations, Simopoulos had been following the work of William Lands and other biochemists who had looked into the ways that omega-6s are processed in human cells. Omega-3s and omega-6s are both essential fatty acids that our bodies need to function and that we must get from our diet. That said, they can lead cells in markedly different chemical directions—so different that Lands describes omega-6s and omega-3s as a kind of Cain and Abel, brothers sharing a common family but inherently competitive. The competition happens on an enzymatic level. If the dominant omega in the blood is omega-6, enzymes will act upon those 6s and form the compounds from arachidonic acid that are pro-inflammatory in nature. If the dominant omegas in the diet are short-chain omega-3s (the kinds found in leafy greens like purslane and spinach) those omega-3s will block the omega-6 pathway and instead lead enzymes to build EPA long-chain omega-3s. And, notably, EPA omega-3 is a proven anti-inflammatory. In other words, a diet rich in leafy greens, pastured animal protein, and seafood will be decidedly less inflammatory than a modern Western diet that is based on soy, corn, and grain/soy-fed animals. Such a diet could even carry with it the tantalizing possibility of *reducing* inflammation.

For physicians like Simopoulos, the omega-6/omega-3 imbalance seemed like a plausible cause for the rise of many Western diseases in the twentieth century. Fat was responsible, just not in the plumbing ways Keys had proposed. Instead, fats were reactive, and different fats reacted in different ways.

This revelation led Simopoulos to try to reconstruct what ancient Mediterranean people might have eaten. Her conclusion was that like the chicken she'd observed plucking purslane, early Mediterranean humans would have eaten a combination of wild field greens high in short-chain ALA fatty acids, seafood with long-chain omega-3s, browsing wild game, olive oil, and only a smattering of grains. All of this would have resulted in an ancient Mediterranean Diet that had an omega-6/omega-3 ratio of about one-to-one.

She suspected that the Cretans and other island Greeks in an unconscious way understood this. But where were they getting the omega-3s in their diet in high enough levels to have an anti-inflammatory effect? In part, she realized, they got it because their bodies, free of the impositions of omega-6s, were more free to elongate vegetable sources of omega-3s. But there was another cultural component. She looked to the traditional Greek way of eating and compared it with other places in the Mediterranean. "Greek Orthodoxy, unlike Catholicism," she told me, "has two fast days. Catholics fast on Fridays. We fast on Wednesdays *and* Fridays. There are 120 fast days in the Greek Orthodox calendar." But a Greek fast is not a total fast. No meat is allowed, of course. No dairy either. Fish is entirely acceptable.

It's important to note here that as soon as one dives into medical research around omega-3s and omega-6s and fats in general, distinct and divergent lines of belief come into sharp relief. The cardiologists, epidemiologists, neurologists, and psychiatrists who embrace omega-3s, many of them serious and legitimate scientists, share a certain commitment to the power of these molecules—a commitment that is, as I would learn later, fervently endorsed by a wide array of alternative health practitioners and supplement manufacturers. Over the course of my research, I came to think of this loose affiliation as "Omega World." It has a certain bold assurance that people outside of Omega World don't subscribe to.

Walter Willett, one of the foremost scholars of the Mediterranean Diet, a professor of epidemiology and nutrition at Harvard T. H. Chan School of Public Health and a professor of medicine at Harvard Medical School, and very much outside of Omega World, downplays the importance of the omega-6/omega-3 ratio. "The idea that the ratio is important," he told me, "is completely fallacious." While Willett doesn't deny that omega-3s are essential, he argues that omega-6s are equally so. "What is important," he told me, "is that you get adequate amounts of both." The really important issues are much larger than simply one omega versus another. What we really want is achieved through a multifactorial life adjustment that includes very limited animal protein, abundant vegetables, high-quality whole grains, appropriate caloric intake, and exercise. Practice this regime and you will go a long way to lowering your risk of heart attack and stroke.

In addition, Willett takes issue with the way later researchers have attacked the original fat research of Ancel Keys ("it's not fair to attack a dead person"). He insists Keys *did* show that *saturated* land animal fat in particular *was* associated with cardiovascular disease but that *total* fat in the diet was not. Willett takes particular issue with authors like Gary Taubes who believe Keys led us down a bad path away from fat altogether and toward an even less healthy path of excessive carbo loading. "The idea that [Keys] pushed a low-fat, high-carb diet is completely wrong," he told me. In even stronger language, Willett's Yale-based coauthor David Katz excoriated the anti-Keys camp in a 2017 white paper. "The thriving cottage industry in revisionist history about Ancel Keys," Katz noted, "may be a product of negligence, ignorance, or even dishonesty. We cannot say which. What we can say, based on primary sources transparent to all, is that the prevailing allegations are false."

This revisionism of the revisionists would come much later. At the height of Omega World's ascendance in the 1980s and '90s, Artemis Simopoulos and an emerging set of clinical nutritionists and dietitians wanted to share what they felt was a hidden secret of the Mediterranean. Simopoulos began organizing an annual conference in Greece timed to the beginning of the Olympic year. She procured funding and flew in thought leaders from around the world to attend discussions on the omega-3s' potential under the thatched latticework of a Peloponnesian arbor. With grapevines intertwined in the trellises above and olive trees surrounding the grounds and the gentle lapping of the sea, who could not be seduced by the joys of the foods eaten by the Greeks for thousands of years? Who could not want to start putting it all into a diet that would reflect that ancient wisdom? Certainly not a young academic from Colorado State College named Loren Cordain. Through Dr. S. Boyd Eaton (one of the originators of the concept of Paleolithic nutrition), Cordain had been invited to attend one of Simopoulos's conferences. After two weeks, the closing meal was more than memorable. "It was just magnificent," Cordain told me. "We had fresh-caught fish cooked in olive oil, fresh vegetables, fresh Greek wine. And that Mediterranean sun was setting. I was thinking, 'It absolutely doesn't get better than this to eat this kind of food with these incredible people.'"

Those long Mediterranean days would stay with Cordain, as would the fresh vegetables and the wild fish. He would reflect at length on his many conversations during the conference and with Artemis Simopoulos's ideas about the eating habits of early Greeks and the ratio of omega-6 fatty acids to omega-3s. He would cross-reference what he'd learned at those talks with the work of Boyd Eaton and other research he'd done into early eating patterns. Eventually he would put it all into a book with a diet concept so catchy he would trademark the name.

He would call it the Paleo Diet.

Whether the omega-3 versus omega-6 hypothesis is true, it is a useful dichotomy when discussing the way civilization and food have changed over time. Balance, whether between omega-3 and omega-6 fatty acids, wild or farmed, or some other set of concerns, does seem to preoccupy early Mediterranean society. But was the balance of food in the preindustrial Mediterranean Diet simply a product of the capacity of a stingy natural environment, or was it a conscious choice? In the five thousand years before the modern Western diet swept over the Mediterranean and began changing its eating patterns, we can see a little bit of both.

In the medical writings from Greek antiquity, a particular obsession with achieving balance starts to arise as hunting gave way to farming. Hippocrates would suggest the idea that the body contained four "humours": blood, phlegm, yellow bile, and black bile. He concluded that "man is never in better health, than when these humours are thoroughly intermingled and at rest, without any one predominating."

And in a way, unconsciously, the ancients did balance the growing omega-3/omega-6 imbalance through a supplement to their normal way of eating. This ur-supplement was my principal reason for coming to Cetara and meeting with Beatrice Ughi.

Once we concluded lunch at Acquapazza, Beatrice marched me down a narrow street to a small storefront bearing the name Nettuno. The door opened onto a large cavernous space, tiled white and redolent with an intriguing smell. On one side of the odiferous spectrum, it bore traces of the watermelon scent a fisherman recognizes as the effervescences of living fish in the water. On the other, it smelled of decomposition and rot.

Beatrice hurried us inside to meet Vincenzo Giordano— Enzo to his friends and intimates. A fine gold chain wended its way through thick hair that cloaked his back and chest.

"*Peccato che non c'è Giulio!*" Beatrice said. "Too bad Giulio is not with us, he's the anchovy ambassador. Enzo manages the production." Enzo led us into the fermenting room and the smell of fish rot hung even heavier in the air.

"This is the only *colatura* production still left in Cetara. Every other place moved up the hill. They got too big. They all moved out. We stayed. We are artisanal." He led us over to a row of *tersigni*, barrels cut into thirds for the specific task of fermenting small batches of the fish sauce made from anchovies.

"Here," Enzo said, "what you have to do is take the fish, and you, well, you pinch the heads off."

"And why, Enzo, do you take the heads off?"

"Otherwise it's"—and here one could see Enzo visibly avoid a less tasteful word of dialect and finally find the Italian—"it's . . . bitter."

He laid out some anchovies, their heads removed, in neat silvery rows. Then a layer of sea salt, then another layer of anchovies. Finally he placed a wooden lid over them, and then he pulled down from a rack a chunk of rock that looked like it could have been prized out of Hadrian's Wall.

"And then?" Beatrice asked.

"And then what?" replied the befuddled Enzo.

"Well, what happens next?"

"Now we wait. For about two years. And then. Colatura."

I saw Beatrice's eyes roll as if to say, "For this I'm paying $100 a liter?" But I also saw her smile and relax. Because, in a way, it was the slow "artisan" process she was paying for. Something that was distinct and treasured as Italy itself.

In fact, though, Enzo's process was not very different from that of the early makers of the original version of colatura that the Romans called *garum*.

Apicius describes the Roman method:

> It is best to take large or small sprats, or failing them, anchovies or horse-mackerel, make a mixture of all and put into a baking trough. Take two pints of salt to the peck of fish and mix well to have the fish impregnated with salt. Leave it for one night, and then put it in an earthenware vessel which you place open in the sun for two to three months [eighteen months for large fish], stirring with a stick at intervals, then take it up, cover it with a lid and store away. Some people add old wine, two pints, to one pint fish.

It is unclear exactly when the various recipes for garum became codified. It is clear from archaeological evidence that its use goes back to the beginning of Bronze Age Mediterranean civilization. The very first distilled fish sauces were probably made in Phoenicia, a nation that predated both Greece and Rome and which perhaps more than any other Mediterranean society based its power and wealth on the sea. In fact if we were to trace the transition from omega-3 societies to omega-6 societies back to early times, Phoenician fish sauce in a way represents that handoff.

A compulsively trade-minded society situated in what is today modern Lebanon, Phoenicia moved goods and ideas from Anatolia to the Strait of Gibraltar. Without Phoenicia, Greece and Rome would have had no written alphabet. The Phoenicians not only invented the letters, but also exported them and endowed the scattered civilizations of the Mediterranean with a way to communicate. It was probably the Phoenicians who began the process of salting fish in mass quantities. It was also they who probably came to understand that whenever you engage in an industrial process there would inevitably be a product and a by-product. The Phoenicians considered the premium product to be salt fish, a commodity that could be shipped throughout the world of the Mediterranean and traded for pretty much anything coming from the land. The by-product was garum.

The Phoenicians brought garum to the far corners of the Mediterranean. As early as the eighth century BCE major fish works were established. The processing installations recently excavated were not unlike Enzo's Nettuno shop in Cetara: a cleaning room, a fermentation room, and a storage room for amphorae. All of these facilities seemed to have two objectives. The first was to create dried, shelf-stable fish products that

could be easily transported and traded for land food throughout the Mediterranean. The second was to process and package the by-product—a liquid that to the modern nose would
probably have a strong smell and an off-putting flavor. Not so
to the ancients. Garum had real value both as a condiment and
later as a kind of supplement.

There was, however, a certain ambivalence about garum in
later Mediterranean societies. The Roman Seneca railed that it
was "the overpriced guts of rotten fish!" Part of the disdain
might have had to do with the overall disdain the Romans felt
for their fish-loving Phoenician enemies: an expression, if you
will, of an omega-6 society's antipathy to an omega-3 civilization. Phoenicia had given birth to the empire of Carthage, a
nation that vied for control of the entire Mediterranean and
was distinctly more maritime than the Romans. Three Punic
Wars ensued between Romans and Carthaginians until the
Romans finally razed Carthage and enslaved its people.

But garum stayed with the Romans. Factories sprang up all
along the Mediterranean coast of Spain and down both sides of
Italy. The Romans imbued garum with all sorts of power, including medicinal, even as they maintained a certain ambivalence about wildness, fish, and the sea.

As ancient society moved toward a cultivated land food
diet, seafood was increasingly seen as a backward way of getting
one's nutrition. For the rising Roman middle class, fish were
associated with poverty and destitution. By the time Rome
reached its zenith of power, it had drifted increasingly away
from wild food. The Romans had standardized the production
of grain in the Nile valley, allowing for the first example of

industrial-scale agriculture in the West. Annual floodwaters from the Ethiopian highlands brought down nutrient-rich soils into a wide swath of the Nile plain. Under Roman control, Egypt became a kind of Iowa for the ancients. In the process they radically changed the environment and the climate of the Mediterranean. Forests were felled, watercourses were redirected for irrigation, and temperatures probably began to rise even as the climate became more arid.

That the development and cultivation of the Mediterranean world were impacting and diminishing ocean and terrestrial wildlife didn't seem to concern the Romans. Only the *uncivilized* people of the ancient world, those who could not figure out the modern technology of earning a living from cultivating land food—only they were reduced to the lowly status of fisherman. "Because they expressed this gap between rich and poor," wrote the classicist Nicholas Purcell, fish "provided the butt for much comic literature." In the end, Purcell concluded, "fish were funny for the Greeks and Romans."

The ancient perception of fish as unserious is also seen in the medical opinions of the time. The Roman physician Galen believed that fish had fewer nutrients than land meat. His exceptions to this rule were grey mullet, sea bass, and red mullet, whose flesh he believed, as the scholar of ancient medicine John Wilkins explained to me, was "closest to human flesh and needs least effort by the body to assimilate it." Galen's belief turns out to be a fairly accurate assessment of the caloric differences of land food meat and fish. One hundred grams of beef contain about 250 calories, whereas a hundred grams of white-fleshed fish like European sea bass contain only about

97 calories. Galen, of course, knew nothing about protein and the fact that fish efficiently delivered it with a minimum of calories. That revelation would be something for later physicians to decode.

Seafood was thus a poor cousin of land food to the ancients, and so fish required some transformative process to win over the finer tables of Rome. Garum was that process—a sophisticated way of bringing the primitive world of seafood into the dining room of the rich. Over time it would also be imbued with powers beyond flavor.

The idea of garum having medicinal possibilities probably originated with the preservative qualities of its high salt content. Egyptian mummies were well salted before storage in their crypts, their preparers believing that a preserved body could be more easily resurrected. When one looks at the nature of garum through a modern lens, the beneficial qualities of salt quickly fall away. Recently Spanish food scientists re-created the process by which Roman garum was made. They found that a group of enzymes naturally occurring within the guts of the fish broke down the component parts of garum into numerous compounds. Standing out among them were omega-3 fatty acids. Garum, it turns out, might have been the first omega-3 supplement.

As Jill Santopietro writes in a recent investigation of ancient fish sauces, it was common practice for Romans to have two teaspoons of garum a day, believing that such a dose contained all the essential nutrients. An agronomist called Columella recommended "pouring garum into the nostrils of sick animals," while Pliny the Elder believed that it had the properties of a laxative when mixed with oil, vinegar, and herbs. Galen prescribed garum cooked with lentils for curing chronic diarrhea. If you should be so unfortunate as to lose your appetite, Pliny suggested garum with garden herbs. Grilled snails could be added to wine and garum to cure an upset stomach.

Mark Kurlansky notes in his book *Salt* that the ancients suggested garum could address a much wider variety of ills, including sciatica, tuberculosis, and migraine headaches. Garum also carried with it a promise of sexual potency. In a first-century CE note, the poet Martial praises his friend Flaccus for developing romantic urges for a girl who slurps down six cups of garum in a row. Other fortifying properties seem to have been attributed to the sauce. Garum and the more plebian sludge scraped from the bottom of the garum barrel, called *muria,* have been found throughout military camps along the Roman campaign trail from Spain all the way to the cold reaches of Vindolanda in Britain. By the time of Apicius, garum was more widely used than salt itself. In Apicius's *De re coquinaria* (what is generally thought of as the most influential cookbook in the ancient world), garum is an ingredient in nearly every one of the roughly five hundred recipes, while salt is mentioned only three times.

The indispensable quality of garum raised its manufacturers up into something much more than just fishmongers. It was said in the ancient world when a child was born under a star at the far end of the constellation Pisces that he would be destined to be not just an ordinary fisherman, but either the catcher of really big fish or, much more profitably, a garum maker.

The archaeological evidence around Cetara bears this out.

Pompeii, just up the road from Cetara, was a hub for fish sauce production and commercialization. The most remembered person from the ruins of Pompeii is not a great leader or a gifted artist but rather a garum maker. Bottles of fish sauce "from the factory of Umbricus Agathopus" turn up again and again in inns, wine shops, food shops, hot drink shops, and homes unearthed from the ancient lava flows.

This, in part, explains the buildup of serious fishing efforts in the Mediterranean during the Roman era. There are various epigrams concerning the quaintness and comedy of fishing scattered throughout the fragments of the ancient world. Some texts suggest that Romans believed fish were more attracted to cooked than to raw meat and that many anglers when they baited a hook would mix bait with fragrant herbs such as rosemary and mint. It was also common (as per Aristotle's suggestion) to place a violinist shoreside to attract skate with music. The fish, hypnotized, would glide into the fisherman's net without resistance.

But by the time of Christ it was not uncommon for a Roman fishing vessel to employ twenty people working nets in a complicated synchronization that was able to take fish big and small. As Roman civilization became increasingly refined and progressively divorced from the essentialness of the sea, the famous sauce that they derived from fish became more important than the fish itself.

For the last part of our time in Cetara, Beatrice and I made our way down to the quays in search of the fisherman who had promised to lead us in pursuit of the fish that was the basis of modern-day garum. As we sat and ate still more anchovies with an afternoon Campari, the captain we were seeking appeared: a dark, heavyset man named Domenico Giordano. Unshaven, with lidded eyes, he looked more tired than anyone I'd ever met in Italy. He had gone to sleep at 5 a.m. and awoken again three hours later.

"So, Captain," Beatrice asked, "are we fishing tonight?"

"Yes," he said, "we're fishing. I don't know if there will be any fish. But we are fishing."

"Why no fish? Are there no fish?" Beatrice asked with alarm.

"Of course there are fish. But I tell you now, the problem is the tuna. They were depleted, but now they're coming back. After the bureaucrats in Brussels kicked us out of the tuna fishery, there are more and more of them. And they're eating all the anchovies."

He of course made no mention that tuna might now be the *only* decently regulated fish in the whole of the sea between the lands. Anchovies, meanwhile, are fished twelve months a year. And the Mediterranean is surrounded by nearly two dozen different nations, each with its own ancient claim on an unrestricted right to use the sea in whatever way it wants to use it; the result is classic tragedy-of-the-commons exploitation. Grudgingly, the sea's various nations have agreed to symbolic actions—a size limit on anchovies to allow the fish to spawn, for example. But with thousands of fishing vessels spread out across the Mediterranean with little in the way of regulation it's hard to imagine the sea being managed sustainably.

In a little while we gathered to board Giordano's vessel, the

Sacro Cuore. Though the sea looked calm and peaceful, the captain was worried about a swell coming out of the west. I popped a Dramamine and advised Beatrice to do the same.

"Why would I take that?" she protested. "It's the Mediterranean!"

We cast off into the inky night, the lights on the hills of the Amalfi Coast bleeding into a dome of stars above so that the rocking of the boat gave one the feeling of being tumbled around inside a giant star-spangled sphere. The only thing that stood out as man-made in the scene was the blazing white cross of the Santuario dell'Avvocata. One of the crew crossed himself and kissed his fingers genuflecting in the direction of the church. Then he settled down on the gunwale and scrolled through his iPhone, periodically kissing the phone when a picture of a favorite saint showed up in his photo stream.

The captain began checking his sonar, and I joined him in the tiny cabin space that served as both wheelhouse and crew quarters. Two narrow bunks piled with blankets and oily rags and newspapers were the only place of repose for the eight-member crew.

I had assumed we would fish in the manner of a typical commercial fishing vessel: we'd locate a school of fish, quickly surround it, and then draw the net tight. The strategy that was actually employed was distinctly geared to a diminished sea. With a thin smattering of anchovies reading on the sonar, the captain signaled the crew and a small dory was pulled up on a crane. The crew's oldest and most feeble member was loaded into the dory and given a rope tied to a boulder. Then the old fisherman was summarily pushed into the sea. The only piece of modern equipment he had was a rickety generator, jerry-rigged to a floodlight. Once he'd pushed himself back from the *Sacro Cuore,* he pulled the starter cord on the generator and the light from the lamps flooded the sea, creating a sapphire dome below the dory that faded to an indigo vanishing point below him. The noise of the generator was deafening, but it didn't seem to bother the old fisherman. He lit a cigarette and stared blankly into the sea. We made a slight jog to the east and then put a second old man in another little dinghy with its own lamp and roaring generator. Then we all sat down to wait while the fish gathered.

Hour by hour, the evening winnowed itself away. The swell built into the early morning hours as the winds started to moan in the stays. It would have been nice to have had a meal made by the two Gennaros or even one of the fresh, sweet figs the colatura maker's wife had given us when we'd left the Nettuno factory. We had nothing and the crew had nothing.

"Fettuccine with asparagus," Beatrice intoned, lying on her back staring at the stars. *"Melanzane parmigiana. Bistecca alla griglia."* She ran through the delicious products of all her producers throughout Italy. She scrolled through Instagram and looked at their various delights. At two in the morning, she pulled herself up and looked at the captain, trying to get a sense of his intentions for ending the long night. The captain answered her inquisitive look with a shrug and returned to the solitude of the wheelhouse and the glow of the sonar.

"Now this," Beatrice said, "is really slow food."

Beatrice had said at the beginning of our time together that when she spoke she was "always on the record," that she had no secrets. But the biggest secret of all was one the Mediterranean had kept from her. Simply put, the balance the Mediterranean promises is too good to be true. Unlike the small plots of land that farmers for millennia have tended with care—blending soil-holding olive trees, nitrogen-fixing chickpeas—no one has ever truly cared about the sea. It has been treated as a mine from which wealth is taken and never returned. At one time, fishing fleets were small and sail powered, lacking in sonar and capable of only a limited range. The Roman writer Oppian describes fishermen in search of small tuna in the Mediterranean deploying "a stout log . . . about a cubit in length" with "abundant lead and many three-pronged spears set close together." The device was dropped through a school of tuna and would come up frequently loaded with fish.

No such device would work this evening. The fleets of the Mediterranean are many and various and the regulations that should limit them go largely unenforced.

But there are also profound changes occurring beyond overfishing. When Egypt dammed the Nile at Aswan in the 1950s, the rich nutrients that once fertilized phytoplankton and prompted them to bloom stopped reaching the sea. On top of that, the yearly cycles of wind and weather have changed, redirecting whole populations of species out of their usual migration routes. In some cases, this is only a geographical adjustment. But more disturbing is a much larger shift, a decoupling, in fact, of the ancient predator/prey relationship that occurs on a microscopic level at the very bottom of the marine food web. The essential relationship of phytoplankton and the zooplankton that feed upon them is changing. Phytoplankton are triggered to bloom by light. As the days grow longer after the winter solstice they increase their numbers. Zooplankton, the first rung up from phytoplankton on the marine food web, are cued by temperature. With waters growing warmer and warmer each year, zooplankton are hatching too early. As a result, both types of plankton, zoo- and phyto-, crash prematurely before juvenile fish, like anchovies, have a chance to feed on them. It is partly for this reason that every year the Mediterranean gets clearer and more beautiful even as it contains less and less life.

An epochal shift is taking place in Mediterranean ecosystems, leading a Yale researcher who conducted dozens of interviews with fishermen all along the Italian coast in the summer of 2015 to conclude that today the average mariner in search of the last wild food can no longer find his way:

> Formerly he would look at Mt. Etna to the east and see the ribbon of clouds that come with the *scirocco*, the southeast wind. Or he would look to the horizon where the sea was a bit choppy and he could see all the way to the Calabrian coast, and know that it is the period of the *tramontana*, the northern wind. Without this, the true meaning of being a fisherman is lost.

The cues nature offers to fishermen are less and less reliable with each passing year. And hence the present technique. A lamp blazing into the water at night simulates an artificial moon. Fish are compelled to venture toward it. It is what fisheries managers call a FAD, or fish aggregating device—a tool that condenses the life of the sea into a small enough area to be fished.

Finally the captain gave the call to haul in. The placid surface of the sea slowly grew alive as the net drew tight and the disparate swimmers came in contact with their fellow fish. When the net had shrunk to about the size of a grade school basketball court the mere brush of the twine against the gathering anchovies caused tiny explosions of scales—showers of fairy dust in the azure water. There is an odd fact about the order Clupeiformes, the order of fish from which most omega-3 oils are harvested: they die incredibly easily. The mere touch of a human hand or a brush with a net cord causes them to let go of their life force in a shimmering instant.

The crew members stared down into the ever-shrinking circle of the net. The odd mackerel zipped back and forth in panic. An "oooo" came when they realized that five or six bonito, smaller members of the tuna family, were also inside. The rest of the catch was incredibly thin. "*Scusi,*" one of the crew members asked me, "how do you say *lavoro senza soldi* in English?" I checked my phone for a translation. "Work without compensation," I read. The fisherman mouthed the words back at me and nodded in agreement.

The Mediterranean, made thin by years upon years of fishing, and thinner still by the damming of the Nile and the rising of water temperatures, was now being strained of its last life, which in turn would be strained and condensed and turned into colatura, modern-day garum. Full of nutrients. Full of life. Full of the fecund richness that the whole of the Mediterranean once possessed.

It is no surprise that today we embrace something called the Mediterranean Diet and the balancing of omega-3 and omega-6 fatty acids that may be part of that diet's strength. But it is a delicate balance that requires a gentle touch on land and a careful eye toward the endurance of the sea. That's not where we're headed. The great secret that Beatrice Ughi did not know and could not tell me is that as the climate warms, the land desiccates, and fisheries fail we are now at a point where the Mediterranean can no longer support the Mediterranean Diet. The depths of the sea between the lands can no longer be passed through humanity's sieve. Other depths in other countries will have to be strained.

Three

THE SUMMIT OF SUPPLEMENTISM

A little while back I learned from an eminent cardiologist that half of all patients first report heart disease to their doctors by dropping dead. No conversation where the physician lays on a tender hand and whispers, "I'm a little worried about your triglycerides." No "honey, you look a little pale today." Just fibrillation followed by abrupt arrest. Boom. Finis.

To date, no one has succeeded at putting a finger on the exact cause of "sudden cardiac death" (as the phenomenon of clutching your chest and croaking on the sidewalk is clinically termed). Is it a chemical imbalance in the body owing to years of bad dietary habits? Is it an electrical short-circuit where the heart fails to get the right signals across misfiring cell membranes? No one quite knows, even though sudden cardiac death is the largest cause of natural mortality in the United States. Into this dark room, where there are many more questions than answers, has sauntered the omega-3.

As I continued to follow the omega-3 around the world, I came to feel that it was somehow bigger than the series of chemical reactions it tempered. That it had a significant role to play in human physiology was clear. But there was also something about the way it behaved in the medical research community that made it seem like a kind of Forrest Gump molecule. If society's obsession happened to be the heart, as it was in the 1970s and '80s, then it was sold on the argument that its role in producing anti-inflammatory compounds makes it worthy as a salve for coronary heart disease. If attention wandered to saving the brain from dementia and growing more neurons for our children, as it has of late, the omega-3 as key to energy transfer across nerve cell membranes was there again. If their structures were famous among chemists for their dynamic changeability, these molecules were also, from a sociological point of view, great Zeligs: they shifted to fit the times.

Because they adapt so well, omega-3s have risen to become one of the world's best-selling nonprescription drugs. Currently, sales of omega-3 supplements and omega-3-supplemented products by some estimates are put at more than $15 billion annually and are predicted to grow at a rate of 7 percent per year for the foreseeable future. And no venue is more indicative of the far-ranging plans the industry has for itself than the next stop on my omega journey, the ground zero of Omega World: the "GOED Exchange," the annual summit of the Global Organization for EPA and DHA Omega-3s.

As my plane circled volcanic Mount Teide and passed over the Canary Islands resort where several hundred businessmen and physicians were gathering for the event, I scanned the odd conference program the organizers had emailed me, with its combination of presentations ranging from gum disease to Alzheimer's to fish oil traceability to motivational speeches on rebranding. All these workshops comprised the culmination of a forty-year-long narrative of positivity. But in the last few years the omega-3 supplement had experienced a significant bump in the road. There was murmuring in the crowd checking in at the Ritz-Carlton that things in Omega World hadn't been this bad since a study had linked omega-3 supplementation to prostate cancer—a charge that many physicians now believe to be discredited. But the studies facing GOED this year cut to the very heart, if you will, of the omega-3 argument. The *Journal of the American Medical Association* had published something called a meta-analysis—a study of studies—that looked at the cardiac benefit of omega-3 supplementation across a range of different criteria. The conclusion? That omega-3 supplementation "was not associated with a lower risk" of cardiac death.

A media feeding frenzy ensued, or at least as much of a frenzy as fish oil can generate—which, actually, come to think of it, is quite a lot. There is no article a journalist on the health beat likes to write more than a good debunking of a miracle cure. A front-page *New York Times* article gathered voices from around the community of doubters, including a physician named Gianni Tognoni who had coauthored a study in the *New England Journal of Medicine* that found fish oil had no beneficial effect on cardiovascular disease. In the article, Tognoni bluntly declared, "I think that the era of fish oil as medication could be considered over now."

Adding to the negative press turn against omega-3s, a documentary episode titled "Supplements and Safety" had just aired on the public television show *Frontline* to high ratings in advance of the conference. (Full disclosure here: when I attended the GOED conference, I was in the middle of filming a different *Frontline* film about seafood with the same director and producer who had made the supplements film.) I'd watched in dismay when the film lingered particularly long on fish oil. At a certain point the correspondent had sniffed a capsule, made a sour face, and then been informed that because omega-3s are such highly reactive compounds, they are prone to oxidation, which means that they rot. A rotten fish oil capsule, the film explained, might actually do more harm than good.

The correspondent went on to interview GOED's preternaturally young-looking executive director, Adam Ismail. In the course of the filmed discussion the reporter nailed him to the floor, asking him over and over again to pinpoint a study that had conclusively proven that omega-3 supplements were effective in treating heart disease. Ismail fumbled, insisting there were many, many studies but in his fluster could not quite make a coherent point. Afterward he would gather his thoughts and point out in the more omega-3-friendly alternative medicine press that "every single meta-analysis of randomized controlled trials (13 in total) that has looked at cardiac death has found a 9 percent to 30 percent statistically significant reduction in risk," and that "the consistency of evidence in this arena is really key because the results are reproduced over and over, but that consistency gets ignored."

Nevertheless, by the time the GOED summit opened in

the Canary Islands, Ismail felt he owed the attendees an accounting. "We all know we've been beaten up over this oxidation topic recently," he said in a mea culpa to the crowd at
GOED's opening session at the Ritz-Carlton.

But in the days ahead, Ismail promised, the vendors of anchovy oil, algae powder, and aquafeed were going to learn a
thing or two about debunking debunkers. There would be
three different talks on the value of non-randomized controlled
trials, which fell outside the purview of the damning *JAMA*
meta-analysis that had caused so much bad press. There would
be a session with two British consultants who had polled the
consumers of omega-3 supplements and promised to reveal
how the users thought about fish oil and what marketers could
do to expand their market.

Most significant to me, though, would be a presentation by
Jørn Dyerberg, the medical researcher who had inadvertently
put omega-3 supplementation in motion. Now a sort of emeri-
tus presence at the conference, Dyerberg is a tall man with a
receding hairline and a playful half smile he offers over the
tops of his glasses; he looks like someone you would want for
your family doctor. Indeed, he is a man with a good heart. He
successfully launched a campaign to eliminate trans fats from
the Danish diet, and at seventy-eight he was still actively
working on many issues that surround cardiovascular disease.
But the heart of his career occurred when Dyerberg traveled as
a young man to Greenland with his supervisor, Dr. Hans Bang,
beginning in 1970. Bang had read an editorial in the *Danish
Medical Journal*, stating that Greenland health records indicated lower rates of cardiac death among the Inuit population.

Scraping together a shoestring budget, Bang and Dyerberg along with a technician named Aase Brøndum Nielson flew to the American air base at Sondre Strømfjord, then boarded a cargo ship and finally a small sailboat that took them from settlement to settlement of this still largely undiscovered country. It had been the great adventure of his life and had caused this very modest and unassuming Dane to take center stage on behalf of a compound that was extremely complicated to explain to the general public.

The story that came out of these journeys remains a sort of foundational myth that today Dyerberg is forced to tell over and over again. On a second occasion, when I talked with him in his lab in Copenhagen, he repeated the story, but with all the keepsakes, medical and sentimental, at hand. A particularly vivid memento was his Greenland diary, as big and as rare as a Gutenberg Bible. He'd had it bound in the skin of a seal one of his Inuit research subjects had shot back in the early 1970s.

"I thought you would find this of interest!" he exclaimed, opening the diary and paging through it with me. "Ah, here you see the young doctor working on his samples. . . . We call that a rye bread motor," he joked, pointing to a picture of himself working a piece of heavy machinery. Since no electricity was available when he and Dr. Bang spun down their blood samples in Greenland, Dyerberg, a typical Dane in his high consumption of rye bread, was that engine.

Contained within the diary was a whole world that no longer existed. Here was Dr. Dyerberg measuring the height of a full-time hunter-gatherer. There were rows and rows of seal carcasses hanging to dry, their fatty blubber the only thing standing between the Inuits and winter starvation. On the next page was a sketch of a dog waiting under an outhouse, ready to scarf down whatever came out of the hole or bite the buttocks of the unsuspecting pooping researcher. Dyerberg chuckled devilishly at the recollection.

"And here," he said, riffling through another ream of papers, "are the original tracings of the blood work." He produced a sheet of yellow graph paper. The tracings showed the levels of the different kinds of lipids in Inuit blood he'd tested. Notable on the graph of the Inuits who had for their whole lives subsisted on a diet of fish, seals, and whales were two sharp peaks. One peak was EPA omega-3 fatty acid; the other was DHA omega-3 fatty acid.

Dyerberg then showed me another set of tracings, this time of the blood work of a resident of Denmark who had been raised eating a typical Western diet of land foods. That chart was mostly flat—no omega-3 peaks for those poor souls.

At the time of his expedition to Greenland, Dyerberg's supervisor didn't even quite know what he wanted to test for. "We had these 130 precious samples of blood," Dyerberg said, growing animated, "the blood from fasting Eskimos up in the northwestern part of Greenland." In twenty more years, their eating habits would start to resemble those of Europe and the United States. "And we thought there'll never be anyone who can do that again . . . so let's do whatever we can! And we decided to do fatty acid analysis. Not because we had a special idea at that time, but just simply to collect the data."

Dyerberg would later tell me that in order to be lucky, you

had to be prepared. In a way, his Scandinavian heritage was the first step in his preparation. Scandinavians, in particular the seafaring Norwegians and Danes, had long been obsessed with marine oils. Before trade incorporated them into the larger commerce of Europe, those dark northern countries were spare places where maximizing the total use of resources— by-products and all—was critical to survival. Beginning with the Vikings, one of the region's most useful by-products was cod liver.

Cod, unlike oily-fleshed anchovies and other hard-swimming schooling fish, have less omega-3-rich red muscle tissue and concentrate omega-3s and other oils in their livers. They then combine this oil with protein to form vitellogenin, which is molecularly tagged and transported to gonads to invest eggs with yolk. Somewhere around 700 CE, Scandinavians discovered that submerging the cod livers in a barrel of seawater caused the oil to detach from the tissues of the organs and float to the surface, where it could then be skimmed off and stored for later use. The naturally concentrated oil became something of a talisman for northerners. Anecdotal observations of patients and cod liver oil throughout the late Renaissance and early Enlightenment seemed to enforce the idea of its goodness.

But merely observing an individual who seems to be improving his or her health after ingesting a substance does not produce evidence of causation. There is no control for other confounding factors and no way to prove whether a factor apart from the studied substance might have contributed to a patient's recovery.

Nevertheless, early versions of what are called association studies did help in the gradual isolation and decoding of essential nutrients across the wide range of the human diet. Association studies are noninterventionist in nature. Groups of individuals who display a given set of behaviors (diet, exercise, and so on) are observed and compared to populations that don't exhibit those behaviors. In modern medicine, association studies are typically an early step that can lead to more rigorous research. But in the early days of medical research they were all that doctors had at their disposal, and they did indeed lead to significant discoveries. It was through association studies with cod liver oil that medical professionals first started to isolate a set of nutrients that proved key to human health.

The first observations of the effects of cod liver oil were linked to a study of a disease that had become increasingly prevalent as the Industrial Revolution spread throughout northern Europe. Malnourished children in sunlight-poor ur-ban slums would often end up bowlegged by adolescence, a condition now known as rickets. The blackening out of the sun in England and the rise of rickets corresponded with the prac-tice of burning sea coal (i.e., coal that washed up on beaches and that tended to produce more fumes than mined coal). During days of particularly poor air quality, Londoners were reported to have "spat black," and as Claire Tomalin writes in her biography of Samuel Pepys, "laundry put out to dry in the open air was soiled again by the dirty air." Slowly, researchers in northern countries pieced the puzzle together and concluded that the disease resulted from a deficiency in vitamin D, which the body naturally generates in the presence of sunlight.

Vitamin D turns out to be stored in high amounts within the liver of cod.

The first part of the nineteenth century was marked by numerous investigations of the efficacy of cod liver oil. The Royal Infirmary in Manchester reported that it appeared to be effective in curing rickets; a physician named Samuel Moore found a similar effect using an ointment derived from shark liver oil. A German study describing a successful five-week course of cod liver oil curing the dreaded disease also helped physicians zero in on fish oil.

Ever more observational studies like these prompted a pharmacist named Peter Möller to standardize the production of cod liver oil. Using a patented chemical process, he arrived at a product that he announced to the world, "didn't taste fishy." Ironically, it took some time to get Scandinavians to accept the new industrially processed oil. As corporate historians of the inheritors of the Peter Möller brand put it, "The consumers of cod liver oil had been used to the fact that 'good medicine must taste bad' and would not believe that the new and better quality was as healthy."

Möller and his advertising team then launched a campaign to institutionalize the regular use of cod liver oil with health claims extending far beyond rickets. The campaign was a success: a spoonful a day became common practice. Fueled by this emerging tendency, Möller built his company into an international presence and died in 1869 with seventy cod liver oil steam factories to his name. That year, Möller's company churned out five thousand barrels of the stuff.

That there is actual medicinal value in cod liver oil has been proven without a doubt. Vitamins D and A contained within cod liver *are* essential for human health. Vitamin D helps the gut absorb calcium and promote bone growth, while vitamin A is critical to vision, the immune system, and reproduction. In underdeveloped countries, where access to nutritious foods is limited, an infusion of those vitamins through whatever means available is worthwhile. The fact that cod liver oil was somehow linked to strong and hardy Vikings further burnished its reputation.

And so by the time Bang and Dyerberg drew blood from their Inuit subjects, there was already a predisposition among Scandinavians to believe that something effective existed within the oil of marine animals. The revelation of the two peaks of EPA and DHA in Inuit blood led them to propose a perfectly logical set of hypotheses: Eskimos have high levels of EPA omega-3 fatty acids and low levels of inflammatory arachidonic acid in their blood. They also have a low incidence of myocardial infarction as well as a slow rate of clotting. Therefore it is possible that "dietary enrichment with EPA will protect against thrombosis." This is a classic example of an association study. While association studies are helpful in determining phenomena worthy of closer, more rigorous examination, they can't really establish causation. As one statistician put it to me, "Association studies will tell you that where there are chickens there will be eggs. But they cannot tell you whether the chicken produced the eggs or the eggs produced the chickens." They may also not necessarily indicate the presence of ducks and geese and whether those two birds influenced the egg laying.

Establishing causation, free of confounding influences,

requires a much more rigorous form of research, one that was first invented to determine the curative properties of common nutrients long before anyone cared to plumb the essential qualities of omega-3s. In 1747 the physician James Lind, sailing aboard a British warship, divided a group of twelve sailors suffering from scurvy into six groups of two. All ate the same diet, but each pair was given a different supplemental potion: one pair got a quart of cider, another an elixir of sulfuric acid, another six spoonfuls of vinegar, another a pint of seawater, still another a spicy paste together with barley water, and finally the lucky last—two oranges and a lemon. These last two men recovered from scurvy within five days, while all the others continued to suffer. This simple experiment has gone down in history as the first control trial, and thanks to it, vitamin C, a key nutrient in citrus fruits, was isolated and correctly termed "essential"—the clinical definition so many omega-3 boosters now desperately want but have yet to receive from national health agencies. Scurvy, a dreaded disease for sailors everywhere, finally had a cure.

Physicians, too, finally had a cure for bias in research: a model for something that came to be called a randomized controlled trial, or RCT. The success of this sort of careful comparative testing would be improved upon in the nineteenth century as a general European scientific movement started to move medicine away from speculation toward science-based analyses of cause and effect. Intimate to that movement was the development of the placebo, from the Latin *placere*, to please; placebos arose from the philosophy of the French doctor Ambroise Paré, who advised that it was the physician's duty to "cure occasionally, relieve often, console always." In other words, doctors are obligated to make their patients feel better even if an actual cure is not forthcoming.

Placebos were famously administered in the eighteenth century by the English physician Alexander Sutherland, mostly for the purpose of placating patients and assuring them that *something* was being done to ease their condition. The British physician John Haygarth took the placebo a step further by using it to unmask bogus cures. In 1799, he used the placebo concept to debunk a common medical device at the time called Perkins tractors. These were metal rods that had the purported ability to draw a disease out of the body. Haygarth swapped in wooden rods for the pricey metal variety and showed that neither had any effect above a certain psychological soothing. He published this finding in a book appropriately titled *On the Imagination as a Cause and as a Cure of Disorders of the Body.*

In the 1920s, researchers further strengthened the impact of placebos by administering them to control groups that were pitted against trial groups receiving actual medication. Researchers like T. C. Graves in *The Lancet* didn't discount the potency of placebos. Rather he saw in them that "a real psycho-therapeutic effect appears to have been produced." Overcoming that power in trials became a primary focus from the 1920s to the 1950s. So intent were they at removing bias that researchers eventually arrived at something called a double-blind study—one in which subjects were grouped at random into placebo and drug groups and where neither the patient nor the researcher knew if the medication being administered was a placebo or not. In this way, antibiotics like streptomycin were established as unequivocal cures for tuberculosis. Over time the randomized, double-blind, placebo-controlled study became the gold standard for testing the efficacy of drugs.

The catch is that such trials are extremely expensive and can take decades to complete. A randomized, double-blind, placebo-controlled trial of omega-3s' efficacy was not applied to Bang and Dyerberg's discoveries until the 1980s. But initial observations were intriguing. One thing the scientists noticed was that when Greenland Inuits suffered bloody noses, the speed at which their blood clotted was significantly slower than it was in westerners, suggesting that omega-3-rich blood had a lower rate of platelet aggregation—a factor associated with reduced heart attacks and strokes (a quality that researchers now attribute to aspirin). When John Vane, later a Nobel Prize–winning pharmacologist, joined with Bang and Dyerberg to follow up on their initial findings, they showed that omega-3s do in fact have the capacity to reduce platelet-coagulating precursors. Together the different strands of research seemed to indicate that omega-3s might be a significant factor in reducing cardiovascular disease.

As sound, solid scientists, Bang and Dyerberg knew what they had found would need to go through randomized controlled trials to be truly valid. There could have been, as always in dietary studies, multiple confounding factors. Greenland Inuits were probably much more physically active than their counterparts in Denmark. Even their diet had confounding factors. In addition to having very high amounts of omega-3 fatty acids in their diets, Greenland Inuits also ate few carbohydrates, a dietary pattern that later researchers have suggested could also have had a cardiovascular effect. In fact Greenland Inuits were in a way early adopters of something now called a ketogenic diet—a high-fat, low-carbohydrate diet that some claim addresses neurological and other disorders.

Outside the scientific community, however, is a nether zone of health obsessives and businesspeople who are ready to grab hold of early, associative evidence. These nonscientists consider an observational study more than sufficient. When a provocative possibility (an end to heart disease) collides with a colorful mythos (Viking traders, Eskimo seal hunters) and powerful market forces (Peter Möller's cod liver oil empire), health-obsessed businesspeople, often Norwegian, charged ahead. And just as with megavitamins, dosages seemed to ramp up to higher and higher amounts. Many of the people I encountered within Omega World suggested a daily dose of two full grams. Quite a pill to swallow.

And so the fish oil business passed from a home remedy to a possible medical curative. Some of the new fish oil supplement business grew out of the traditional cod liver oil industry that Möller had created. But it also drew its raw material from the most far-flung reaches of Norway's marine manifest destiny. In the eighty years preceding the emergence of omega-3 supplements, Norwegians built a financial empire from the reduction of the whales that roamed the Southern Ocean. When large-scale whale-oil refining ended, Norwegians continued to try to figure out how they might make use of the resources Antarctica and the Southern Ocean had to offer. And, curiously, that switch has driven them back to the very food whales depend upon: krill. Krill is now one of the most expensive ingredients used for omega-3 supplements. In 2016, I asked Hallvard Muri, then the acting director of the largest Norwegian krill harvester in the Antarctic, why they had chosen to set up a multimillion-dollar operation in one of the most inhospitable seas in the world.

"Really the important thing about the krill," Muri told me, "is that when you take the krill oil you don't have this fishy aftertaste."

"Fishy aftertaste?"

He went on to explain that because krill oil is composed largely of phospholipids, compounds that resemble the fat configuration of human cell membranes, krill oil could be more easily absorbed and incorporated into human cells. If this was the case, then one needn't take the 1,000-milligram fish oil horse pill some of the more exuberant embracers of omega-3s were recommending. They could instead take a tiny pill, red from the natural astaxanthin that would also shield the oil inside from oxidation. A smaller pill meant less actual oil in the human stomach and, then again, less chance of a fishy burp.

Fishy burps aside, the 1980s and '90s were marked by researchers trying to isolate what it was exactly that omega-3 fatty acids were doing in the human body. Some followed Ancel Keys's old cholesterol theory, thinking that perhaps serum cholesterol might be lowered by a daily fish oil dose. Bill Connor, a doctor working out of Oregon, went so far as to put twelve patients through a trial in which every subject was asked to eat a salmon steak for breakfast, lunch, and dinner along with 45 to 90 milliliters of salmon oil every day for four weeks—around twenty-five times the dose that even the most ardent GOED members administered to themselves. "At first people were real excited about the prospect of eating all that salmon," Connor's widow recalled to me a few years ago, "but after a while, you know . . ."

Certain subjects became convinced that they were actually beginning to smell fishy, and Connor, upon hearing this, called over his student Bill Harris and asked him, "How would you like to run a little sub-experiment?" Connor had Harris buy twenty pairs of long underwear and asked the trial subjects to wear them for twenty-four hours. Harris then took the under-wear and cooked it in an acetone bath to extract the lipids. No fish oil was detected. It was all a trick of the mind.

A similar trick of the mind happened with cholesterol as well. At the conclusion of Connor's salmon trial, most subjects were found to have a notable decline in serum cholesterol. But later trials found that it was not omega-3s themselves that were lowering subjects' cholesterol, but rather the absence of other dietary elements, red meat and dairy in particular, that *raises* serum cholesterol. In other words, it was as Harvard's Walter Willett had said: reducing saturated fats from land food meat and dairy in one's diet is the real game changer.

But neutral or negative results haven't to date slowed the supplement industry. Throughout the 1980s, fish oil capsules were marketed as a means to lower cholesterol. After numerous clinical trials confirmed that cholesterol levels were unaffected by fish oil, the federal government weighed in. In 1992, the FDA noted that positive cardiovascular effects applied "only to

the consumption of fish" and that "the data from clinical studies revealed that omega-3 fatty acids had no effect on serum
cholesterol, LDL cholesterol, or HDL cholesterol, the blood
lipid variables most closely associated with risk of Cardiac
Heart Disease."

And so today, the marketers of fish oil pills have moved the
goalposts to more abstract concepts, with "inflammation" being the key word. Today inflammation is the affliction that a
certain wing of the medical community constantly invokes
much in the same way an earlier generation invoked cholesterol
as the villain in our veins.

In a summary of all of inflammation's incarnations in the
present medical era, the physician and writer Jerome Groopman noted that the National Institutes of Health now consid-
ers inflammation a "research priority" worthy of hundreds of
millions of dollars. The journal *Science* devoted an entire 2013
issue to inflammation. As Groopman summarized in *The
New Yorker:*

> In best-selling books and on television and radio talk
> shows, threads of research are woven into cure-all tales in
> which inflammation is responsible for nearly every mal-
> ady, and its defeat is the secret to health and longevity.
> New diets will counter the inflammation simmering in
> your gut and restore your mental equilibrium. Anti-
> inflammatory supplements will lift your depression and
> ameliorate autism. Certain drugs will tamp down the si-
> lent inflammation that degrades your tissues, improving

your health and extending your life. Everything, and everyone, is inflamed.

Though Groopman's tone here is a bit tongue in cheek, physicians *do* see inflammation as an extremely important and perplexing problem—just the kind of confusing situation that is profitable territory for supplement companies. So marketers of supplements have joined the medical community in obsessing over inflammation too. The only problem here is that something like 30 percent of the thousands of proteins that circulate in our cells have something to do with inflammation. Omega-3s surely play a role in some of those interactions, but it's hard to say unequivocally whether it's a starring role or just a bit part.

One would think that all of the many qualifiers that temper whether cardiovascular disease may be addressed by omega-3s would give someone considering an omega-3 pill cause for skepticism. But the rise of omega-3s as one of America's most popular dietary supplements coincides almost exactly with a concerted and ultimately successful effort by the $37 billion supplement industry to escape government-required clinical trials.

Until the 1970s, the United States had been making halting but steady progress in codifying and regulating pharmaceuticals. This edifying process began as an effort to stamp out various phony snake oil–like treatments, including actual snake oil. In the late 1800s a traveling cowboy-huckster named Clark Stanley claimed to have traveled to Walpi, Arizona, so that he

might see the Hopi Indians' snake dance. There he purport-
edly swapped his Colt revolver for a two-year residency with
the tribe's medicine man and later returned to civilization to
market Clark Stanley's Snake Oil Liniment. As Dan Hurley
relates in his excellent history of the supplement industry, *Natural Causes*, Stanley would tour the country in full cowboy re-
galia and conduct a show in which he would kill a pair of
venomous snakes before a live audience, draw out the rare oil,
and mix it with nine other oils in what he said in court testi-
mony was "a big glass jar like you make orangeade in." At the
show's conclusion Stanley would sell the freshly made potion
alongside hundreds of bottles of a previously manufactured
product that was described as a "liniment that penetrates muscle, membrane and tissue to the very bone itself." When the
U.S. Department of Agriculture began a fraud investigation
into Stanley's concoction, chemical analysis revealed that his
snake oil wasn't even made out of snake oil. "The sample con-
sists principally of a light mineral oil," the USDA concluded,
"mixed with about one percent of fatty oil, probably beef fat,
capsicum and possibly a trace of camphor and turpentine."

Findings like these led to the 1906 Pure Food and Drug
Act, which sped the creation of the U.S. Food and Drug Administration. Subsequent amendments strengthened the FDA
and led the United States toward a more rational and less magical way of understanding medicine. By the 1960s, America
fully embraced the tedious and expensive philosophy of randomized, double-blind, placebo-controlled trials. In 1972,
however, just as Jørn Dyerberg and Hans Bang were setting

out for Greenland, another scientist with two Nobel Prizes to his name set medical research back a hundred years.

Linus Pauling is credited with some of the key discoveries that led to the eventual decoding of DNA. By the early 1970s, though, his career was in decline and he had begun to fade from the public spotlight. It was then that Pauling took up the cause of vitamin C, claiming that supersized doses could counteract a wide range of illnesses from the common cold to cancer. Pauling's bizarre recommendation of 3,000 milligrams a day (fifty times the recommended daily allowance at that time) finally caused the FDA to take notice and seek to limit vitamin dosages to below one and a half times the recommended daily allowance. The supplement industry perceived the dosage limitation as a direct threat to their business model. And so in 1976 a consortium of supplement makers pushed through the U.S. Senate what came to be called the Proxmire Amendment. An FDA chief counsel later called the legislation the most humiliating defeat in the history of the agency. And even though its immediate effect was only to prohibit the FDA from regulating dosage limits of megavitamins it opened the door for the supplement industry to much more robustly defend itself. A defense that one legislator was particularly enthusiastic to mount.

Utah senator Orrin Hatch had put himself through college going door to door selling vitamins, and early on he became a good congressional friend to the supplement industry. With Hatch at the helm, the 1994 Dietary Supplement Health and Education Act created what Dan Hurley called "a third hermaphroditic category" that was neither food nor drug. This new category was effectively sealed off from control by both the food side of federal regulation and the drug side. Now supplement makers could put whatever they wanted in a capsule and sell it as a supplement. No science or evidence of any kind was necessary.

Meanwhile, during the same period, legitimate research became considerably corrupted by forces outside the traditional medical establishment. While the Pure Food and Drug Act of 1906 had created scientific norms for medications before they could reach the general public, over the course of the twentieth century the idealism of that era was outpaced by a race for profits. A medical study in its pure sense is a way of seeking knowledge. But once medical trials start to take their principal cues from industry, research becomes marketing. Objective science actually proves this. In a meta-analysis of forty-eight medical papers that comprised thousands of individual trials, the outspoken medical watchdog Peter Gøtzsche found that industry-sponsored studies more often had favorable efficacy results, favorable harms results, and favorable conclusions for the drug or medical devices of interest compared with nonindustry-sponsored studies. You get what you pay for.

And so when I left Jørn Dyerberg at the GOED conference and wandered back into the main auditorium, it was with conflicted feelings. On the one hand, I wanted Dr. Dyerberg's findings to be true. I trusted him as a real scientist and believed his intentions were sound and his methods cautious. The conference, however, was clearly dominated by those who were there to make money. And since all of the negative results from recent clinical trials had started to stem the flow of money into manufacturer's coffers, a kind of public soul searching of the omega-3 industry was occurring. Something that was immediately apparent when a pair of marketing specialists took the stage at the GOED conference.

Judy Taylor had been hired by the BASF corporation, one of the world's largest producers of omega-3 ingredients to survey several thousand omega-3 supplement users. She was later joined onstage by her British colleague Gill Ereaut, and together they laid out how the consumer had come to think of omega-3 supplements. As Taylor paced the stage of the conference she laid out what she called "The Life-Health Journey" of the individuals in her survey: a prevailing narrative about how the respondents felt about their health at various ages and how that narrative could be probed for profitability.

"Up until the age of about twenty everybody does believe they're immortal," Taylor said, but that starts to change. "Your first baby, at about thirty, or your first stiff knee . . . is where you start to think about [your finite life span]" and you begin to plateau. By thirty-five you realize that you are on a "declining slope," and by forty-five you are in crisis. You can see the decline ahead of you, but for the group that is dedicated to omega-3s, it's all about desperately trying to limit that decline and "make that plateau extend."

If the arc of life went according to the plan of the most ardent supplement users, that plateau would continue well into a person's eighties and then a quick drop-off would occur; shortly thereafter a sudden death would come with little suffering for the moribund and a minimal amount of collateral damage to loved ones. That plateau and the hopeful extension of it Taylor and Ereaut later referred to as "the Indian Summer of life." My ears perked up. Herein lay the essence of the omega-3 pitch: the marketers of supplements were suggesting that they could transform the rind of life into an Indian summer.

Desperate to avoid a feeble old age, Taylor explained, different people responded in different ways—in four ways, actually—to the realization of this newfound vulnernability. There were the "Redeemers": people who had lived horribly unhealthy lives, "who had pushed it too far," and they knew it. The sorts of people who had partied too hard and sought redemption, who wanted to be reborn. Next there were the "Preventers": people who were serious and measured in their approach, who seemed to have been focused on a long healthy life from the very start. There were also the "Hopefuls"—people, usually women, who were prone to binge on any new product and had a tendency to "believe in magic," but who were not likely to stick to a regimen in order to try the new, best thing.

But from a marketing point of view, the most valuable group was the "Disciples." They have dipped into the science as much as their science-light education allowed them to. And in so doing Taylor noted that they "have found proof"—so much so that if you asked them to stop taking their omega-3 supplements for ten days just to see what would happen, they would refuse.

The omega-3 "disciples," Taylor went on to say, sought "harmony," "control," and "better functionality." They were "health orchestrators" who thought of themselves as "extraordinary people" who could control their lives and lengthen the odds on dying. If you could get the Disciples on board, there was real market potential. Or as Taylor put it, "It's here that you ladder up . . . to powerful, emotional spaces about immortality and invincibility," all based on the high, professional, "pioneering science," with the primary message that omega-3s are "extending valuable life."

It occurred to me as I listened to her explain the mind-set of these rational health orchestrators that there was something about their reasoning that had little or nothing to do with science. Yes, their hope was somewhat science based. But many of these hopes were abstract. Real science didn't promise increased vitality through omega-3 supplementation. What omega-3s offered from a clinical standpoint was a reduced risk of dying of cardiovascular disease. The only moment when you would finally be able to prove that omega-3s did in fact extend that plateau of useful life would occur when you lay on your deathbed at a very advanced age and expired peacefully with minimal suffering. To believe in that positive end of life wasn't really science. It was faith.

Taylor concluded her presentation with an image that incorporated all of the many vague feelings about omega-3 supplements that she felt could help the brand. The image was of a sleek female form, not young exactly, but in excellent physical condition. In the place of her legs the artists had inserted a DNA-ish double helix spinning downward and fading away from her backside into infinity. From her torso an aurora borealis splayed upward and spread through her parted arms into a gesture Taylor indicated was meant to imply reincarnation.

It was in this hybrid creature, this half-human, half-helix, that I understood the awkward position the omega-3 now holds. The compound is no doubt a critical part of evolutionary history and a necessary part of the human diet. Objective science has shown it to be one part of regulating inflammation and inflammation's inverse resolution; and there is no question that omega-3s are an integral part of the nervous system. But it is something of a leap of faith to go from observing physiological functions of omega-3s in the heart and the brain to recommending a supplementation of two grams a day.

Magical thinking has long pervaded the public's perception of medicine. Of the handful of medical papyri surviving from ancient Egypt, most are largely based in magic. Only one set, the so-called Edwin Smith papyrus, is a thoughtful treatise that follows illness in a very evidence-based way from diagnosis to appropriate treatment. Still, it's the magical ones that seem to have held the most weight. Medicine is the last thing standing between life and death, and so we imbue it with messianic powers. The most important struggle of medicine through its five-thousand-year history is to rid itself of magic—to use the power of the scientific method to arrive at conclusive, objective truths.

The uneasy coexistence of science and the hope of magic explains why many people today continue to be confused about what exactly medicine can and cannot do for them. On the one hand, the apparently miraculous breakthroughs in nutrition and pharmacology that took place in the nineteenth and twentieth centuries give a sense of incredible, almost mystical power. But those breakthroughs were made possible only by randomized controlled trials. It was this objective, painstaking science that brought us remarkable discoveries like vitamin D for rickets and penicillin for bacterial infection. Through those fundamental discoveries and innovations a large swath of preventable deaths were indeed prevented, leaving the door open to the possibility that perhaps many other causes of decline and death were equally preventable. But on the other hand, as medicine advances into increasingly more complicated syndromes with multiple pathologies and afflictions like dementia and cancer, medical science of late seems to be providing diminishing returns. We might not see another magical-seeming breakthrough like penicillin in our lifetimes.

And so the public's relationship to medical science is a mishmash of unrealistic hope and profound disappointment. As an editor at *The New York Times* once put it to me, the public perceives science "as a machine that turns incoming data into foolproof conclusions that any honest scientist will accept as the truth." In fact, the everyday practice of science is always an argument. When the public sees that scientists disagree, they become disillusioned and worry that something sinister is going on. But there's nothing sinister at all. Honest disagreement is an integral part of science.

Which brings me to a presentation at the GOED conference on the nature of scientific investigation itself. GOED had invited a statistician named Michelle Wiest to lead the room in a discussion of randomized controlled trials and meta-analyses, how they work, and what we can and cannot infer from their findings. She would also present a case study, an analysis of none other than the Rizos *JAMA* study that had found no significant effect of omega-3s on cardiovascular disease.

She began by saying that thirty years ago, almost no one cared about meta-analyses. These "studies of studies" are a defense against the rising tide of research investigations, which have relentlessly multiplied since Dr. Dyerberg first journeyed to Greenland. Part of the reason for this increase is the expansion and diversification of legitimate research. But a large part of the increase is a plague of phony journals that have taken root on the internet. Some journals charge a fee to underpublished scientists looking to rack up easy credits. Others plug pharmaceuticals. Still others may be part of a larger web traffic scheme. Whatever their motivation, fake journals have become so persistent and irritating to researchers that some real scientists have taken to baiting them with their own bogus creations. In 2015, a fed-up group of Polish scientists invented an imaginary editor named Anna Olga Szust (derived from the Polish word for "fraud") and offered her online with the thinnest of academic credentials. Fifty different fraudulent academic journals invited Dr. Fraud to be an editor.

Meta-analyses are designed to cut through all that chaff. The scientists who conduct them establish criteria by which many different studies and entire journals can be discarded. Then with whatever remains they seek to derive larger trends that reveal broader truths. Also, since meta-analyses combine the results of many studies, they vastly increase the sample size—something statisticians consider to be more robust and closer to those ever-elusive absolute truths.

Phony journals weren't the subject of Wiest's talk at GOED that morning. Rather, she wanted to show how authors look at many different legitimate studies and reach conclusions about a general trend in the different data. Walking through the steps of a sound meta-analysis, she noted that there is an inherent bias built into all meta-analyses of published studies. Why? Because nobody wants to publish a study where nothing happened. Except, of course, when you have something to debunk. And here, perhaps within the *JAMA* meta-analysis of omega-3s and cardiovascular disease, lay something of an agenda—the eternal academic desire to be noticed. For if the authors could show the startling news that omega-3s didn't have a significant effect on preventing cardiovascular disease, the world would take an interest. By combining the trial results from twenty different studies, the Rizos et al. authors concluded that the P value, the measure of compatibility between observed data and the hypothesized absence of an association between omega-3s and cardiovascular disease, was large. Translation: the meta-analyses suggested that omega-3s had no real impact on cardiovascular disease. Wiest, as best as she could, tried to offer different ways of interpreting that conclusion while hundreds of Omega World eyeballs glared at her from the audience. "Making these hard-and-fast decisions based on P values . . . is very arbitrary," she said. "Statistics is not mathematics. It's a very subjective art." Whereas the *JAMA* study's authors had concluded no effect of significance, Wiest thought there was "evidence of a small effect of omega-3 fatty acids on the prevention of cardiac death." At the end of the day the effect seemed to people outside the world of statistics quite minimal. By taking a fish oil pill on a daily basis, the Rizos *JAMA* study estimated that the risk of cardiac death decreased by 1 percent.

This conclusion has produced a divide in the medical community and the nonmedical people embroiled in its debates. The anti-omega-3 camp, often hailing from the distracted and headline-driven world of journalism, failed to delve deeply into the *JAMA* meta-analysis data or the methodology used to determine "significance." Later, when I asked Martina Pavlicova, a biostatistician at Columbia University, to offer her objective opinion, she found much to ponder in Rizos et al. She questioned the *JAMA* authors' decision to lump together four studied outcomes—all-cause mortality, cardiac death, general sudden death, and stroke/heart attack—as well as their conclusion of no significance from that aggregation of outcomes. In addition, she sensed a potential distortion in the way the authors double-assessed each outcome using two different methodologies. The result was that the somewhat significant effect on cardiac death was drowned out, like a lone alto singing in a choir of tenors. Since Rizos et al. effectively doubled the number of tenors in the choir, the voice of the one significant alto grew even fainter. "If they were testing ONLY cardiac death," Pavlicova concluded, "they would find the cardiac death significantly associated with omega-3s. So, saying that they had nonsignificant finding overall but highlighting only cardiac death is making the study sound more focused and rigid than it was." And we must also remember that we're not really talking about tenors and altos here. We're talking about life and death. A 1 percent protection in risk from cardiac death, one of the most common natural causes of mortality in the United States, translates into thousands of lives saved.

Furthermore, the anti-omega-3 camp would not examine the other bodies of evidence out there. They would discount the retrospective association studies on individuals (like Dyerberg and his Eskimos) that seem to show a relationship between omega-3 consumption and reduced risk of death. A 2016 meta-analysis of these kinds of association studies in the journal *Nature,* for example, showed an overall 6 percent decrease in all-cause mortality by taking omega-3 supplements. This meta-analysis included more than five times as many subjects and much longer time frames than the *JAMA* randomized controlled trial meta-analysis. But because it was a meta-analysis of association studies, not a survey of randomized controlled trials, the anti-omega-3 camp did not consider it relevant.

The anti-omega-3 camp might also fail to mention that several confounding factors have entered into the epidemiological data since the early and very positive omega-3 studies of the 1980s and '90s. The most significant is the use of statins, a set of anti-inflammatory compounds derived from Japanese mushrooms. Statins have a proven effect backed up by extremely expensive trials. Since one of the main things that omega-3s do is reduce inflammation, statins might have solved the problem before omega-3s got a chance to work on it. In fact, there has never really been a large randomized controlled trial of "normal people" and omega-3s; to date, trials have focused on people who are already being treated for cardiovascular disease. Indeed, one of the reasons why the first trials of

fish oil in the 1980s showed such promise was that those subjects didn't have the wide range of cardiovascular treatments at
their disposal at that time. The more recent disappointing trials, meanwhile, were all carried out in the context of much
more sophisticated cardiovascular therapies.

Another key issue that is not taken into account by the anti-
omega-3 camp is that the randomized controlled trials to date
have generally not tried to establish a baseline for omega-3
blood lipid content in subjects before trials began. There does
seem to be an associative relationship between high omega-3
blood lipid levels and lower rates of fatal coronary heart disease. So the lack of a demonstrable effect may simply be due to
the fact that patients could have already achieved a level of
protection outside the trial. Those adhering to a Mediterranean Diet would have the added benefit of having an omega-6/
omega-3 ratio that might better mitigate inflammation.

The GOED meeting drew to a close. A final dinner was
staged in a banana plantation with a table that stretched
three hundred yards through a thicket of tropical fronds. It was
clear that the participants had found the conference to be an
uplifting show of solidarity. Supported by their mutual confi-
dence, they had banished doubt from the halls of the Ritz-
Carlton, and the growth of the industry, after a small post-*JAMA*
hiccup, seemed assured.

At the closing session of the meeting, Jørn Dyerberg was
brought onstage and asked to give his thoughts on how the
industry might proceed into this rosy future. He promised he

would "not tell the old Eskimo story again" and instead offered
some exciting new research he'd come across in preparation for
his talk. He paused, furrowed his brow, and read the next slide:

"Effect of Fish Oil Encapsulates Incorporation on the
Physical, Chemical, and Sensory Properties of . . .
COOKIES!"

Even Dyerberg, it seemed, felt that research into omega-3s
sometimes ventured into some pretty odd territory. Laughter
filled the gathering, accompanied by smirks that acknowl-
edged the often unacknowledged fear at the GOED conference: that the omega-3 phenomenon flirted dangerously with
jumping the shark.

But as he moved on and scrolled through multiple slides of
studies demonstrating the positive effects of omega-3s on cancer, macular degeneration, cognitive function, all of the many
fields that his visit to Greenland had birthed, you could not
deny that Dyerberg still had an unbridled enthusiasm for these
molecules. He was excited that finally, huge "megabucks"
studies were underway. These new studies would be robust,
randomized controlled trials commissioned by serious institutions. What got Dyerberg particularly excited was the VITAL
study at Boston's Brigham and Women's Hospital: 25,874 participants for six years ingesting acres upon acres of fish oil capsules. A study that would at last test fish oil's effect on people
not already suffering from cardiovascular disease, that might
finally determine whether or not the average Joe should keep
on taking his fish oil pill.

That study was published in the fall of 2018, two years after I'd spent my weekend in the Canary Islands with the luminaries of Omega World. There was much fanfare in advance of its publication. Its authors kept their cards close to their chests until the results were finally revealed at the annual conference of the American Heart Association.

For members of Omega World, the findings were disappointing.

The tantalizing hypothesis that omega-3 supplements might decrease the risk of developing several forms of cancer was unequivocally shot down. With regard to heart health, the VITAL study showed that omega-3 supplements did not have a robust effect on reducing cardiovascular disease. There was a notable downtick in heart attacks, primarily among subjects who reported low intake of fish in their diet—an outcome that suggests that most of us can get the benefits of omega-3s as part of a balanced diet. Across the thousands of participants and a variety of cardiovascular outcomes, however, the study's authors could not make a sweeping, overarching conclusion about the positive effects of omega-3 supplementation. The industry came away without the silver bullet they'd hoped would advance the golden pill.

Four

THE REPUBLIC
OF REDUCTIONISM

I left the Canary Islands and the thirty thousand omega-3 studies in a muddle.

The thing is, I liked the people of Omega World—the scientists and dietitians, the pill manufacturers and the fish oil refiners. The part of me that had always wanted fish to be more significant felt an allegiance to them. In all the journalistic sniping at Dyerberg's findings in recent years I sensed a modern echo of what the classicist Nicholas Purcell had written about ancient impressions of seafood: "Fish were funny for the Greeks and Romans." This mocking, this relegation of the ocean to a sad little corner of discourse and diet made me want to protest. "No, fish are not funny!" I wanted to cry out. "They're important!"

And so everything I heard in the Canary Islands was appealing. The GOED speakers had "found proof" and it was more comforting to fall back on that version of the truth than it was to play the role of the pesky journalist, pointing out this inconclusive *JAMA* study or that murky randomized control trial. It was uncomfortable mentioning to Dr. Dyerberg (and then feeling his ire) that a Canadian scientist had gone back through the Greenland public health data and concluded that rates of cardiovascular disease among Inuits might not have been as low as Bang and Dyerberg had originally found. It was easier to cite as evidence all the instances where omega-3s appeared in evolutionary history and the Forrest Gumpian way they turned up in so many different parts of human physiology.

But as much as I wanted to believe in omega-3s-as-medicine, there was another side of the story that suggested the presence of a second agenda in the fish oil debate—a kind of ghost limb that worked the machinery but never quite showed itself. In fact, while the fish oil supplement business seems like a big deal, it turns out to be just a sheen over the surface of a much deeper pond. For long before omega-3 supplements became so popular, an industry arose that used the same omega-3-rich creatures—not for medicine, but for an odd array of agricultural and industrial purposes. Ultimately, it was this reduction industry that created the oily fish extraction system that now consumes millions of tons of marine wildlife every year. Today, one in every four fish caught on earth is "reduced" into oil and meal and used for agriculture, land animal husbandry, and, most recently, fish farming or "aquaculture." To fully understand reductionism and all the dynamics that shaped its rise one must head south, below the equator, to the home of the largest single-species fishery in the world—to the onetime Inca kingdom now called Peru.

. . .

A fishery is defined as the combined presence of a commercially exploitable species and the fishermen who do the exploiting. The particular species that makes such a huge presence of fishermen possible in Peru is *Engraulis ringens*, also known as the Peruvian anchoveta. During the last half century anywhere from two to twelve million metric tons of anchoveta have been caught off Peru every year—oftentimes more than the tonnage of *all* fish and shellfish caught annually in U.S. waters.

Peruvian anchoveta are so abundant because of something called an upwelling. Upwellings occur throughout the world, and though they account for only 1 percent of the ocean's area, they are where nearly half of all fish in the world are caught. The Peruvian anchoveta's upwelling is the planet's largest and is bordered by land with high, steeply inclined mountains. When wind hits these impassable coastal mountains, it is directed offshore, and as it barrels east to west across the sea it pushes a warm upper layer of water farther and farther away from the coast. With the warm water ceiling removed, cooler water rises to take its place. Omega-3-rich phytoplankton along with deepwater nutrients rise with that cooler water. When the plankton rise, they encounter sunlight. Photosynthesis and mitosis do their work, and soon a green bloom carpets the first layers of the ocean. The abundance of forage triggers zooplankton to bloom and feast upon the phytoplankton. When the Peruvian anchoveta finally hatch, they feast upon that zooplankton abundance. And with that abundance come humans to harvest the fish.

Anchoveta lie at a strategic juncture in the marine food chain. Below them are solar-driven plankton. Above them are higher predators like tuna and whales that require fish flesh to survive. If the anchoveta are removed from between these two biological layers, there is no way for the solar energy gathered by plankton to pass up to the higher rungs of the food web. Remove forage fish like anchoveta from their critical juncture and you get a much simpler, more primitive system. Other species of small, oily fish play the same important energy transfer role in many different ecosystems around the world: herring for cod in the Gulf of Maine, menhaden for striped bass in the Chesapeake, sardines for bluefin tuna in the Bay of Biscay.

By traveling to Peru at what should have been the height of the anchoveta season in mid-October, I was hoping to see this food web in all its glory. But as I started planning my trip, that abundance was called into question.

2015 was a year with an unusually intense El Niño, and in such times the typically boisterous activity of upwelling eco-systems are dialed back to a whisper. A cycle linked in part to solar activity causes the hot air that normally blows offshore to linger over nearshore waters. The air grows stagnant and stale and the offshore breeze poops out. Instead of moving offshore, warm water lingers and acts like a hot lid on a crypt. Cool wa-ter and the nutrients within it never find the light they need to allow phytoplankton to bloom. The zooplankton starve and fail. The anchoveta go into lockdown mode and barely repro-duce. And the fishermen—well, until fairly recently, the fish-ermen just kept on fishing.

In the weeks before I departed for Peru, the likelihood of an opening to the anchoveta fishery shifted daily. IMARPE, the Peruvian fisheries research agency, had conducted assessments of juvenile anchoveta and indicated that there weren't enough fish in the water to allow the boats to have a go at them. A minimum of five million metric tons would have to be provably present for fishing to begin, and so far only two million could be accounted for.

Just as it seemed as if the anchoveta season would be canceled, IMARPE sent out another research vessel and declared that in fact, yes, people could go fishing. Judging from everything I'd seen from how fisheries typically work, it seemed rushed. Patricia Majluf, a onetime Peruvian minister of fisheries, now the vice president of the environmental NGO Oceana Peru, told me that she believed that all the counting and recounting was simply the anchoveta industry forcing the issue. Like a player at a craps table, they were rolling the dice again and again until they got the number they wanted.

The thought bothered me as I boarded a LAN Chile flight for Peru. Again it played in my mind when I woke from a fitful sleep the next morning as the plane descended over Lima, a sprawling cut-rate Los Angeles where instead of a film industry a multibillion-dollar reduction industry thrived. The principal activity of this industry, now present on every continent on earth, is the transformation of the flesh of fish into a powdery substance called fish meal or fish flour, which is in turn fed to a variety of domesticated animals. The oil, once burned off as a waste product, is now refined and either used for aquaculture or, most recently, for dietary supplements.

Soon after landing, I found my interpreter and driver and headed up a highway that skirted a rambling coastal desert. On either side of the road, dunes had been thrown up by an awesomely powerful wind, a wind so strong that it caused our van to teeter on its wheels. And then all at once the car was enveloped in a putridity that made me gag—the smell of millions of anchovies being boiled down to meal and oil. I tucked my nose into my shirt and felt a wave of nausea rising.

"Ah, that's nothing," my interpreter said. "You used to be able to smell Chimbote from like thirty kilometers away. When I was a kid and traveling with my family we used to say, 'Roll up the windows, here comes Chimbote!'"

We arrived quayside and found our boat, a red-and-white affair called the *Maricielo*—"the sea and sky." We clambered aboard and took up our positions in the fading warmth of early evening. The boat started and headed toward the open sea. Only about a quarter of a mile into the journey, though, the captain gave a signal to shut down the engines.

"Why? Why can't we go fishing?" I asked.

"We have to wait for the other boats," the captain said.

"Why? If we go now we'll really get the fish! We'll get there first!"

"Believe me," the captain said, "we don't want to get there first. If we get there first—ay yay yay."

I reached around in the darkness and found a slightly soft place on the deck that turned out to be a coil of arm-thick rope. It was padded enough for a kind of sleep. The running lights were turned off, and slowly my eyes grew accustomed to the moonlight. One by one, a series of white islands came into view. At first I thought their intense whiteness was only an afterglow on the retina after a day of driving through blazing sand dunes. As I adjusted to the twilight I realized that that intensity of white was quite real. Because the islands turned out to be cloaked in yards-deep accumulations of bird poop.

To some extent the story of the Peruvian anchoveta, and the greater story of reductionism, is a story of bird feces—or, more precisely, soil fertility and the degree to which humanity has wasted it. Long before people sought anchoveta for its omega-3 oil to put into fishmeal and fish oil capsules, they pursued anchoveta in its processed form—a form that came out of the other end of a seabird as guano.

That Peru would come to be known for its guano was a hard fall from its Inca days of glory. Conquistadors had originally come to the country in search of gold and silver. When Pizarro captured the last Inca king, Atahualpa, the king offered to fill a giant room with a mountain of gold and then to refill it two times over with mountains of silver in exchange for not getting burned at the stake. The chief made good on his promise and duly filled the rooms with treasure. Pizarro showed his gratitude by sparing Atahualpa the roasting stake and having him strangled instead. Once the king was gone, the country was emptied of its silver and gold until the most valuable thing that remained was guano. An entire archipelago of poop-strewn islands stretching to the north and south of the capital. Eighty-four islands and countless other smaller poop rocks. Guano as far as the eye could see.

But this was no ordinary feces. This was excrement that to the failing soils of postcolonial America and Europe was worth its weight in gold.

The so-called guano islands off Chimbote and elsewhere down the Peruvian coast are the result of extensive nesting colonies of Inca terns, cormorants, petrels, penguins, pelicans, and other seabirds that feed on anchoveta. In some areas the guano reached a depth of thirty feet. Though the Incas occasionally dipped a toe into it and used it to fertilize the nearby land, the guano islands were ignored until Peru landed itself in bankruptcy. In 1845, Ramón Castilla became the first popularly elected president of Peru and found the country in a deep hole of debt. But there was no gold and silver left to pay down that debt. Only bird poop.

Fortunately for Peru, another kind of debt was afflicting the rest of the world that made all that bird poop quite valuable. After decades of intensive growing of corn and wheat, the soils of the Northern Hemisphere were giving out. The initial fertility bonanza settlers experienced after breaking the primeval Great Plains sod was waning. For a while, the American land productivity was propped up by the ongoing transformation of Great Plains wildlife into fertilizer. In grade school textbooks, we read about the pioneers and cowboys who laid low the hordes of bison that roamed the plains. We never read about the mop-up operation that came after the bloody campaigns were over, the processors who specialized in making use of all the dead and dying that were left. It was these odiferous entrepreneurs who made a second fortune off all that destruction. Bison bones were a hindrance to tilling soil and became a source of income for poor homesteaders of the Great Plains, who were paid to collect them for the reduction factories. Carcass by carcass, the skulls and bones of the buffalo were ground down into fertilizer. But that too would give out, and eventually the great powers of the global north would turn to the south to try to revitalize their lands.

The contributions of an adventurous and quirky scientist named Alexander von Humboldt would help pave the way for the great inter-hemispheric poop trade. Born in 1782 to a wealthy Prussian family, Humboldt blew through his family fortune exploring the world and building a reputation as the foremost naturalist of his era. He was one of the principal vehicles through which the world of the nineteenth century came to understand scientific investigation. No one quite like him exists today—a hugely charismatic figure who was both rock-star famous and profoundly serious and rigorous as a researcher. Much of western Europe fell into the thrall of rational scientific inquiry because of Humboldt and his many adventures. With laughably inadequate clothing and primitive climbing equipment, he scaled some of South America's highest peaks. He came excruciatingly close to describing a theory of evolution. (Darwin would carry Humboldt's seven-volume *Personal Narrative* with him aboard the *Beagle* and would note that "my admiration of his famous personal narrative, part of which I almost know by heart . . . determined me to travel.") Along with persuading Darwin to pursue a line toward evolution, Humboldt was also the first to foresee how land food production hastened deforestation and caused acute local climate change.

Most relevant to the anchoveta story, Humboldt was to

discover and promote the concept of isotherms—lines along which temperature is constant often regardless of latitude. Isotherms offered a means of mapping the way the ocean flowed and by extension how fish traveled and where you might find them in greatest abundance. His name was given to one of the world's most important isotherms, the Humboldt Current, which flows from Tierra del Fuego north past the westerly bulge of South America where Peru and Chile meet. It's this isotherm that helps distribute nutrients to the upwelling that feeds all of those Peruvian anchoveta.

Humboldt's life was intertwined more directly with Peruvian anchoveta too: It was he who brought the guano islands to the attention of Europe. Though he had little care for money, many of Humboldt's inquiries later made great profits for others. He had a habit of collecting piles of samples from South America's plains and jungles and mailing them back to European experts for analysis. He was amazed by the endlessly deep stores of guano off Chimbote and sent a packet of it to a renowned chemist named Humphrey Davy. Just as the vitamin researchers of the day were starting to break down the world of food into essential nutrients, Davy was doing the same for plants, concluding that fertilizers provided a set of essential minerals that help foster plant growth. He quickly saw that the nitrogen (in the form of ammonia) and phosphorus the Peruvian guano contained could do much toward getting crops to increase their yields. Humboldt would never see a dime from his discovery, but the people who made use of guano would make a killing.

The great Peruvian guano secret got out, and soon crews were mining it day and night. Giant vessels were constructed whose sole purpose was the global hauling of bird droppings. In the course of researching this book I discovered that the nearly four-hundred-foot-long vessel *Peking* that sat moldering at the easterly border of my Manhattan neighborhood in the South Street Seaport was in fact a guano ship. Once upon a time, it was fitting to send such a spectacular boat south for poop.

With guano harvesting came collateral ecological damage. Bird nesting areas were blasted away by the poop miners, and the baby birds were fed to the workers. Shells of the destroyed eggs were ground and used as mortar to build out the city of Lima.

Meanwhile, by the mid-nineteenth century the guano wealth of Peru became so important to the United States and other Western powers that warships were frequently sent to Peru to ensure its safe passage to the buyers in the north. When the Peruvian government tried to gain greater control over the resource, American leaders raged at their impudence.

But the export of guano would have other reverberations that would echo back to fish. Ten thousand miles to the north of Peru, along the American eastern seaboard, farmers were tired of paying for all that South American guano to prop up their exhausted soils. The time was ripe for an alternative. That alternative turned out to be an extremely common but seldom-used fish called menhaden.

In 1792, a Long Island farmer wrote in a local newspaper that he had learned from Native Americans that menhaden was particularly good as fertilizer. By 1811, Americans were taking that advice a step further by boiling menhaden on the shores of Rhode Island at makeshift camps. The true industrialization of the fish happened a bit later. One early story from 1850 relates how a Mrs. John Bartlett from Blue Hill, Maine, came into the store of one Eben B. Phillips with a "sample of oil which she had skimmed from the kettle in boiling menhaden for her hens." She told the oil merchant that menhaden were abundant all summer near shore and were easily processed. Once the oil was pressed from the fish, the remaining meal could be used to fertilize fields, much in the same way as Peruvian guano. Upon receiving a promise of $11 per barrel, Mrs. Bartlett returned to Maine and produced thirteen barrels that summer. Soon menhaden processing plants were built throughout New England and the mid-Atlantic. The new fish oil barons hailed the industry's development as the antidote to South American guano tyranny.

Reductionism rapidly became a driving force in the development of fisheries in the United States, with menhaden leading the way. Though it's hard to imagine today's trendy Long Island Hamptons as putrid fish death camps, the hulks of the old menhaden processing plants that can still be found on those shores attest to how thoroughly the industry dominated New York's fine sandy coasts.

At the same time a parallel reductionism was rising in Europe, primarily in Scandinavia. In the late 1800s multiple herring oil factories were established along the Norwegian coastline. Norway didn't get a large-scale electricity grid until the 1950s, and so herring literally brought Norwegians out of the dark—particularly important in a country mired in long nights for much of its high-latitude winter. Still brighter lights were to come from herring. Throughout the twentieth century Norwegians used herring and other fish oil to make nitroglycerine—a key element in explosives. Militarily, the substance was so important that the very first offensive action the British took after the Dunkirk disaster during World War II was to sneak over to Nazi-controlled Norway and blow up a series of fish oil plants on the remote Lofoten Islands. In peacetime, reductionism helped grow Norway's animal husbandry. Since only 3 percent of Norway's land was suitable for agriculture, the fishmeal left over after the oil was extracted was a boon to the growers of livestock. With fish as feed at their disposal, Norwegians could grow many more tons of land animal protein than the pasture of their spare land could normally support.

It is hard, I know, to drum up sympathy for all these little, oily fish converted into so many tons of meal and gallons of oil. But it's important to remember that in the nineteenth and twentieth centuries nothing was safe from the cookers and the fertilizer plants—not even the largest and most intelligent creatures in the sea. Indeed, it was whales that strengthened and solidified the economic position of reductionists and drove the market in new and odd directions.

The common impression is that whales were hunted only in the Moby Dick days, pursued for oil used to light lamps. But the lamp oil era of whaling died with Herman Melville, and by the turn of the nineteenth century whaling itself was poised to go extinct. In fact, by the time the largest schools of whales ever seen were discovered off Antarctica, whale oil had very little practical purpose. Petroleum had displaced its role as a provider of light. Menhaden oil had displaced its role as a solvent and lubricant.

That all changed in 1902 when a German chemist named Wilhelm Normann invented a process called hydrogenation. To hydrogenate a fat, the dynamic double carbon bonds that make fatty acids like omega-3's so useful to living organisms are blasted with hydrogen atoms in the presence of a catalyst. The resulting fat is much more stable and, equally important, melts at a much higher temperature. Thanks to hydrogenation liquid oil could be transformed into transportable bricks of margarine.

Shelf-stable margarine quickly became a primary way fats got into the Western human diet. Margarine was particularly popular during the cholesterol scare of the 1960s—highly ironic given that today researchers believe that trans fats correlate with cardiovascular disease more strongly than the fats in the butter they were replacing. The American Heart Association now identifies trans fats as a significant factor in heart disease since they do double damage both by lowering good (HDL) cholesterol and raising bad (LDL) cholesterol. None of this was known at the time of margarine's invention. The only problem anyone could find with it was the fickleness of the international oil market. When the most popular oil crop, linseed, declined by a third in 1900, Antarctic whales proved to be an economically viable substitute.

With a purpose in place for the wholesale slaughter of the great southern whales, an industry began to take shape. Who would do the slaughtering? A political development made Norway the prime candidate. Just as hydrogenation was being perfected, Norway was completing a century-long independence project, finally breaking away from Sweden in 1905. Historically a whaling nation, a newly liberated Norway was in desperate need of capital. With an abundant supply of margarine-producing blue, finback, and humpback whales there for the taking, and with no legitimate national jurisdiction to regulate the fishery, the Norwegians quickly established what would become one of the most infernal slaughterhouses in history.

The scenes of depravity witnessed by many of the early whalers defied imagination. As D. Graham Burnett relates in his epic history *The Sounding of the Whale,* a kind of ever-churning Hades transformed the intelligent bearers of healthy polyunsaturated fats into trans fats in a soul-searing way. Workers encountered horrifying whaling stations where blubber-filleting flensers climbed up carcasses "like mountaineers, cutting steps up the flesh as footholds for their boots." Processing plants that reeked like "charnel houses boiling wholesale in Vaseline" posed grisly dangers such as a rotting mother whale's "forcible ejection of an unborn fetus (which could be larger than an automobile)." Such scenes led the most hardened whalers to remark, "What penalty, I used to wonder, would the gods in due time inflict for such a sacrilege?"

The Norwegian government had little sentimentality about whales. Even though Antarctica is about as far from Norway as any two points on earth can be from one another, Norwegian national identity came to be tied up in the spoils of the white continent. Because of their long history in processing cod liver oil, the Norwegians already had the market sense to work the whale blubber trade. The profits from the country's main whaling station in Grytviken on the island of South Georgia were stunning even by dot-com standards, bearing dividends of 15 and 32 percent respectively for 1907 and 1908. The sheer magnitude of the undertaking was also startling. From 1911 until the whaling moratorium of 1986, the population of Southern Hemisphere blue whales alone collapsed from an estimated four hundred thousand individuals to fewer than two thousand lonely remnants. Other species suffered similar devastation.

At a certain point output was no longer measured in terms of numbers of creatures killed but in BWUs—blue whale units, or the amount of oil that could be rendered from one blue whale carcass. A fin whale was about three-quarters of a BWU; a humpback, one-quarter. And though talk would arise periodically within Norwegian fishing circles of establishing "maximum sustainable yields" for cetaceans, the overall numbers of whales in the Southern Ocean only went down. In the early part of the twentieth century, the British mathematician Colin Clark determined that if all the whales of the Southern Ocean had been killed and reduced to oil in one fell swoop and converted to liquid capital, the annual return on investment would be significantly higher than the value of a smaller, sustainable harvest made year after year. With such monstrous economics working against it, it's clear that whalers and whales had little chance for coexistence.

But even more mad profit was to be made, in particular from the extensive waste that piled in the wake of primary processing. Tons and tons of *skrott*, the leftover stripped carcasses of the whales, were typically set adrift, befouling the air and sea for miles. Soon the whalers saw the error of their ways in even more profit: the refuse itself, if boiled, turned out to account for another 30 percent more oil. What was left after the boiling was also eventually valuable. The market opened up by Peruvian guano meant that all of that whale skrott, bones and all, could be put to good use. In this way the bodies that housed the great minds of the sea were erased from the bottom of the world.

Whales were only one phase of a larger move toward reductionism. In the United States, the profits from whales and menhaden no doubt inspired West Coast companies to begin developing reduction businesses of their own. Whereas the eastern menhaden companies used a fish that was never considered food, the Californians turned to something that they had been working hard at considerable cost to transform into high culinary fare.

The California sardine, similar in evolutionary provenance to the anchoveta and also rich in omega-3 fatty acids, had been an object of exploitation since the late nineteenth century. Though occasionally companies would label those sardines as mackerel (the preferred oily fish of the day), they were accepted in their own right and favorably compared with the French canned sardines produced from the fish of the Mediterranean. But then reductionism entered the picture.

In the 1880s and '90s, when the business began ramping up, the boiling down of sardines on the West Coast was just a side business, the repurposing of the industrial by-product of sardines that were being used for human consumption. But sardines are famously bony. The knifework involved is meticulous and grueling, and the best workers needed to be highly skilled. Paying them a decent wage was unavoidable. Companies that didn't want to waste all that money on skilled labor found that throwing a whole fish into a fertilizer cooker was much more cost-effective. So, like the menhaden before it, the California sardine became yet another target for reductionism.

Regulators who were forward thinking enough to see where a wasteful culture of reductionism could lead tried desperately to create some kind of disincentive for the practice. Eventually, fisheries legislation with an almost moral tone emerged. For two decades beginning in 1920, the California Department of Fish and Game passed laws declaring that whole fish could not be used for reduction. "Canned sardines," wrote the U.S. Bureau of Fisheries, "must sell at a price that is based on their own cost of production. Production of fish meal and oil cannot continue to dominate canning." In other words, good, nutritious fish must be used to feed humans first. Only the leftovers were to be thrown into the fertilizer cookers. The endlessly inventive reductionists countered by lowering the price of canned sardines below the cost of production. Why would anyone want to sell something for less than it cost to make? Simple, really: the fish were much more valuable as fertilizer than as food. The reductionists fixed the price of canned sardines so low in order to move them out of the way quickly and focus on the truly lucrative business of reducing life into dust and grease.

This tension between product and by-product is a surprisingly prevalent theme in the history of food systems. One could argue it began with garum and salted fish back in classical times. But it continues, especially in the age of supplements. Whey protein, a waste by-product of cheese production, today can be as valuable as cheese. Chicken feathers and carcasses can sometimes compete with chicken flesh in price because feed companies can turn them into valuable nutrients and float them on the volatile animal feed commodities markets. And so it was in California. The reductionists even produced a brand of higher-quality boneless sardine products specifically because it generated even more waste for reduction.

In time, reductionists would come up with even more cynical ways to stay ahead of regulators. In 1926 a Monterey canning company towed the processing barge *Perulta* outside of U.S. territorial waters and thus outside the legal jurisdiction of regulators. Eventually, every major sardine port from San Diego to San Francisco was host to offshore processing barges that churned and burned the clupeid wealth of the California coast into dust.

By the 1940s the California sardine would collapse. This was due in part to a climate event that warmed water temperatures. A strong shift in the solar cycle known as the Pacific Decadal Oscillation in 1941 altered the planktonic structure of the fishing grounds. Like El Niño, the Decadal Oscillation is a sine curve of temperature variation, driven in large part by ocean gyres. In warmer temperatures, sardines prosper. When the water cools, anchovies take hold. But when environmental conditions shifted from a sardine regime to an anchovy regime in 1941, no significant corresponding decrease in fishing was mandated. A natural trough in the sardine population was dug even deeper when fishing continued unimpeded, and when the fishery completely collapsed, millions of dollars' worth of ships and processing equipment were idled.

It was at that point that reductionists started their exodus from California in search of more promising waters abroad. One American named Sal Ferrante, an experienced canner and reduction plant owner, sold his entire processing plant, which was then dismantled and shipped to South Africa to exploit forage fish along that country's western shore. When the new owners reconstructed the old plant in South Africa, it looked and functioned exactly as it had in California. The front door even bore the same name: Ferrante & Co. Meanwhile, Ferrante himself kept on the move. He picked up and moved to Peru, where he helped launch an industry even larger than those in California and South Africa. Indeed, reductionism ratcheted up everywhere during the 1950s and '60s. In Norway, the original homeland of whale-based reductionism, the industry grew to such an extent that by the late 1960s, 95 percent of the fresh pelagic fish caught in the country were reduced for animal feed and fertilizer. The Norwegian reductionist experiment expanded far across the Atlantic, targeting a fish called the Atlantic capelin, the primary forage for Grand Banks cod. By the 1980s codfish populations had collapsed from Newfoundland to the Gulf of Maine.

Peruvian anchoveta fishing grew apace. By 1970 the fishery had grown into a major national industry, and eventually one in every five fish caught in all the oceans of the world was a Peruvian anchoveta.

Which is how I found myself curled up on a coil of rope on the *Maricielo* under a starry dome behind a guano island in the churning Pacific. Around two in the morning, I was jostled awake by a crew member and realized that we were under way. I pulled myself up and in the gloaming started to make out a boat to our starboard. And then another, and another. And a half dozen—wait, no, *two* dozen—vessels off to the port. I looked back starboard side and saw I had been mistaken, that there were three dozen boats, and then—actually, there were too many boats to count. They were everywhere, all cruising in the darkness toward some invisible goal.

I joined the captain in the wheelhouse. He was a man exactly my age but with many more years on his lined face. He squinted with a weariness beyond weariness—so tired that he wasn't tired—into the sonar. As the engines slowed I heard a desperate sad moan come out of the darkness.

Arggghhuphhhhh
   Mwaaaahahahaha

"What is that sound?" I asked.

"*Lobos de mare*," the captain said. Sea wolves in their language, sea lions in ours. The Spanish expression seemed much more applicable to the mobbing packs circling the boat. From the darkness still a louder, stronger chorus.

Arggghhuphhhhh
  Mwaaaahahahaha

"How many are out there?"
"So, so many. So many you can't even count them."
The boat churned, the sea wolves wailed louder and louder.

Arggghhuphhhhh
  Mwaaaahahahaha

I lay back on the coil of rope and shut my eyes. Only seconds seemed to pass, but suddenly I felt a hand on my shoulder waking me up and a shout. "*Listo!*" Ready. The captain called out a string of numbers over the radio, then others in the fleet answered back with numbers of their own. The sonar beeped repeatedly and urgently, as if it were crying out, "Fish! fish! Oh, so many fish!" A man wearing a T-shirt bearing the word OMEGA called out another string of numbers—some internal code for what the eight men aboard had to do to make a mile of net shoot out from the transom of the boat.

A cry went up, "Ayyyyy!" Suddenly the boat reared back on a wave and shifted in the wind, and the thousands of feet of net were on the wrong side of the boat, threatening to capsize the whole endeavor. Sea lions chuffed and wailed. The boat lurched again, and suddenly *ping!* the net was free and whizzing toward the dark horizon.

The crew raced right and left, jumping like ballet dancers over the snaking lines. A pod of dolphins shot in from port, trying to intercept the school before they could enter the net, but the men had already started to draw in their catch. The man in the OMEGA shirt whistled three times, and the ropes began hauling in on a giant block and tackle that dangled over the crew like an executioner's ax.

As the haul continued and the sun bled out over the top of the horizon, I looked up to see that the sky was black with birds. Petrels, gannets, cormorants, Inca terns, all those birds that made all those islands of feces, turned and whirled and plunged like a relentless attacking squadron down toward the anchoveta. Turning from the birds to the net, I saw no fewer than three dozen sea lions. And on either side of us there were some forty boats, each with its own forty sea lions. That's why we'd waited for the fleet, I realized. If we'd gone out alone, we'd have lost all of our fish to the roving packs.

All around the net the sea lions frolicked. In the Greenpeace photos of fishermen confronting marine mammals, you often see the poor sea lion swept up in a sprawl of net, drowning because of it. Here the sea lions knew exactly how to work the system. Ecology teaches us that successful predators strive to never expend more energy in the hunting than what they will acquire from the spoils of the hunt. The sea lions watched the net tighten and waited for the fish to concentrate, and when they decided that the humans had made the anchoveta into an appropriately dense and deliciously oily ball, they actually jumped *into* the net. The crew shouted and cursed and tried to get them out, but they resolutely refused.

"They are being nice to the sea lions because we're here," my interpreter told me. "If we weren't here . . ."

And as if to fill in his ellipsis, *bang bang bang* went a gun from the deck of a nearby vessel.

Finally, the net drew tight. One by one the fat sea lions slipped out of their own accord, like obese waddling patrons who have overstayed their welcome at an all-you-can-eat buffet. Two refused to budge. They raised their noses and gestured their chins at the crew as if to say, "How can I possibly leave all this fatty deliciousness?" The crew shouted and bellowed and cajoled and finally the last pair gave up and slipped out—imagine a pole vaulter, five hundred pounds too heavy, struggling to slough his body over the bar. Then the anchoveta came in: a giant ball of silver energy. This haul was orders upon orders of magnitude larger than all the hauls of all the anchovies I had seen in the Mediterranean. In a single pull we'd just landed two thousand pounds.

It all seemed so unfathomably abundant, such a rich expansive vision of the way the natural world should be. I had to keep pinching myself and reminding myself of what I knew: that it was possible that I was looking at a remnant. Just as the Inca king Atahualpa filled Pizarro's room once with gold and twice with silver before being sent to his grave, so too has the Peruvian upwelling filled the coffers of the foreign industrialists, first with guano and then again and again with fish. The quantity of what remains is disputable. During the buildup of the anchoveta industry in the 1950s, '60s, and '70s, the Peruvian shorebird population and the once-valuable guano they created plummeted from forty-five million birds and 330,000 tons of guano to fewer than seven million birds and 50,000 tons of guano.

Take away the anchoveta and you take away the birds. Take away the anchoveta and you take away the sea lions.

Since the 1970s, when the Peruvian anchoveta fishery crashed due to overfishing combined with an El Niño event, conditions have improved. Like many fisheries around the world that had been overexploited in the postwar buildup of fishing fleets, the pursuit of anchoveta was transformed in the 1980s and '90s to a "limited entry fishery" where quotas were established. Once upon a time, anyone with a boat could go out and fish. Now there are strict limits in place that curtail the numbers of boats fishing and the amount of fish each boat can catch. There is no more race for fish, no rush to empty out the sea before someone else empties it underneath your nose. Just a reliable yearly removal of a portion of the fish with the hope that it will refill again the following year. And even though all of these anchoveta would indeed make perfectly good food for humans, the reduction industry asserts that in spite of attempts to market anchoveta to people, humans don't seem to want to eat them. As Andrew Mallison, director general of the International Fishmeal and Fish Oil Organisation, put it to me, "If there's no human demand to satisfy, why, if this abundance of fish is in the ocean and it can be harvested sustainably . . . why *not* extract some value from it?"

But beyond this question, there are larger questions about the purpose of any living organism. Beyond profit, is reductionism the most ecologically and environmentally efficient use for a quarter of the world's wild fish catch? What would the world be like if reductionism didn't exist? We know, for example, that Peru was once encouraged by the United States to export large amounts of tuna to strengthen the backbone of the Allied troops overseas during World War II. We know that all those tuna certainly ate anchovies. And we now know that the tuna industry has shifted away from South America to more distant shores. We know that codfish on the Grand Banks and in the Gulf of Maine plummeted not long after reductionism went after capelin and herring in the North Atlantic. We know that declines in northeastern gamefish like striped bass and weakfish occurred more or less concurrently with the reductionist pursuit of menhaden from Maine to the Chesapeake Bay. All of the higher-level marine predators we like to eat depend upon an almost unimaginably large forage base to maintain numbers capable of supporting commercial fisheries. When we catch and reduce twenty-five million tons of prey, does it not inevitably have a cascading effect on valuable predators everywhere?

But perhaps the most maddening thing about reductionism is the way it aids and abets the very same land food agriculture that is causing so many problems for fish in so many other places. This is particularly true when it comes to the historical use of anchoveta for livestock production.

As the author Michael Pollan explained in his *New York Times* investigation of the contemporary beef industry, up until the mid-twentieth century the majority of the livestock humans raised grazed on pasture. When animals are fed on an all-grass diet, they don't require much in the way of additional nutrients. Starting around 1950, however, farmers realized that they could bring pigs, chickens, and cattle to market much more quickly if they were fed corn and restricted to high-density "concentrated animal feeding operations," or CAFOs. A corn-fed CAFO cow reaches a market weight of twelve hundred pounds in as little as fourteen months, whereas the same growth for a pasture-raised animal can take three years. The production cost for pasture-fed animals is roughly double that of industrial feedlot meat, which any visitor to a high-end grocery story can see reflected in the retail price. But while grain feeding is extremely cost-effective for farmers, it is extremely calorie inefficient for the world. As a recent report from the Natural Resources Defense Council notes, "If all of the crop production currently allocated to animal feed were directly consumed by humans, global food production would *increase* by some two billion tons and food calories would increase by forty-nine percent."

In addition, transitioning grazing animals to a high-energy, nutrient-poor diet based on corn has health consequences for livestock. But it turns out that fish, whose flesh contains not only omega-3s but also protein and a host of other amino acids, can act as nutritional compensation for the dietary elements grazing animals lose when they are removed from pasture and put on corn. It is for this reason that export-driven reductionism in Peru rose in lockstep with the rise in American animal confinement.

All of this was hastened by dire economic conditions in Peru. In 1968, Juan Velasco Alvarado led a revolution that completely upended the old Castilian agricultural system. Landowners were stripped of their property in the hope that the country's poor could share the profits of the once top-heavy system. The economy became state run. International investors were kicked out. But nationalization didn't do much for food production. Soon, the country was starving. With no other way to bring in much-needed foreign currency, the revolutionary government turned to anchoveta and specifically the production of fishmeal. During this tumultuous period, Peru provided 45 percent of the world's fishmeal supplies, much of it going to animal feed.

Confined American chickens took particularly well to fishmeal. At first, scientists called the fishmeal effect on chickens the "unknown growth factor," but later they found that anchoveta had a unique fatty acid composition that increased poultry efficiency. Then came pigs. One of the chief ways that DHA omega-3 fatty acids form mammalian brains is by passing via mother's milk to infants during nursing. As CAFO pork production increased into the 1970s and '80s and farmers lost patience with the inefficiency of nursing piglets the old-fashioned way, they found that fish oil added to piglet formula could help weaning proceed more quickly. Pregnant sows fed fishmeal also gave birth to bigger, healthier litters. Soon millions of tons of little fish were being eaten by pigs.

But whether it is pigs or chickens that are now roped into the corn-and-soy-plus-supplement feed structure, one thing is immediately apparent from a health perspective: feedlot meat is markedly lower in omega-3 content than that of pasture-raised animals. A meta-analysis of 196 papers on milk and 67 papers on meat showed omega-3 levels to be about 46 percent higher in grass-fed animals than in industrially raised, grain-fed animals.

But beyond agriculture reductionism has found still more markets. Pet ownership in the United States ramped up throughout the second half of the twentieth century to the point when now 68 percent of homes have pets, far in excess of the proportion of households with children. Pet ownership grew hand in glove with feedlot meat consumption in the United States. As industrial slaughterhouses arose to accommodate all the meat Americans wanted to eat, a shadow industry developed in its wake. Today forty-seven billion pounds of raw animal material waste is rendered down into eighteen billion pounds of products a year, and about half of that is pet food. Since shareholder wealth is ultimately based on growth, the makers of pet food were forever trying to expand their market. Ralston Purina advertised heavily, especially after World War II, promoting the idea that "happy family life required pets."

The great maw of the renderers was at first indiscriminate. According to a 2004 report to the U.S. Congress, animals for rendering could come from as diverse sources as roadkill and "downers" (the industry term for cattle that can no longer walk). In all, according to the National Renderers Association (does *every* profession get a trade association?), there are something like 250 rendering plants operating in the United States.

Business is business and profit is profit, even in rendering pet food from waste ingredients. As the pet food industry expanded throughout the 1960s and '70s and slaughterhouses became increasingly efficient at carving meat down to the bone, pet food manufacturers began substituting cheaper corn and soy for meat. This was fine for dogs, but cats were a different story. The problem turned out to be an amino acid called taurine, something found only in animal flesh. Fish, though, are particularly high in taurine. Enter the anchoveta once again.

Today the U.S. pet food industry is worth over $24 billion. The number one trend in contemporary pet food, according to industry analysts, is "premiumization"—the development of specialty high-end foods that please those consumers who want to treat their pets as human children. "Premium" pet food makers thus avoid some of the nation's less appealing source material. Just as in premium human food, premium pet food producers focus on natural and organic ingredients.

The wild Peruvian anchoveta is both.

I stepped off the gunwales of the *Maricielo* reeking of anchoveta slime but pressed on farther to even smellier environs. Eventually I arrived at one of the many anchoveta plants owned by TASA, the world's largest producer of fishmeal and oil. Lined up at the quays were two piers stretching a quarter mile into the sea. Berthing on one side, anchoveta fishermen were unloading their catches. On the other, transport ships were preparing to disembark for the wider world. Today, as the grinders and boilers of anchoveta look for still another way to use all of this product, the latest and most profitable market turns out to be fish farming in China.

In the last half century Chinese aquaculture has grown

from a cottage industry to a centrally planned behemoth that now grows more than half of the world's farmed fish. Even though many of the fish China grows are vegetarian fish like carp and tilapia, which don't convey many omega-3s to the people who eventually eat them, the fish themselves grow nearly twice as fast when they are fed a diet high in fish oil—a diet they would never encounter in the wild.

So strategically important is anchoveta to the Chinese seafood economy that just before I visited Peru, the China Fishery Group acquired Copeinca, a Norwegian corporation that until recently controlled a major portion of the anchoveta trade. Soon after, China Fishery went bankrupt, in part due to poor anchovy fishing the year of my visit. But Chinese companies continue to circle this little fish, trying to figure out how to keep a secure stake for the future of their aquaculture industry. Other major mergers between aquaculture interests and reduction fisheries have taken place recently. In October 2017, Cooke Aquaculture, one of the largest growers of salmon in the world, acquired the menhaden fishing company Omega Protein for $500 million.

In a way, I suppose, aquaculture's interest in reductionism shouldn't be that objectionable. In the fish farming scenario, at least fish are eating other fish. And as a recent analysis out of Canada's Dalhousie University pointed out, Peruvian anchoveta can be one of the most low-carbon foods on the planet. The midwater trawls used to capture anchoveta produce little drag on vessels, keeping fuel consumption to a minimum. The problem is that the reducers don't view anchoveta as a standalone species. They view it as an ingredient to be blended with other ingredients. And most feed for popular species like salmon carries a familiar set of components: soy and other carbon-intensive row crops.

When I was finally able to sit down to talk about all this with Humberto Speziani, the TASA senior management adviser who oversaw the dozens of anchoveta reduction plants, I was surprised to learn that he had mulled over all of this as much as I had. I had expected to find in Speziani a coldhearted capitalist, the Great Reducer himself. Instead what I found was a thoughtful man who really did contemplate the impact his industry had on the environment and on the huge challenge we face in trying to feed what will soon be nine billion people. He was a kindly bald grandfather of a man who warmly patted my shoulder as we spoke. He had a thick but endearing accent and gamely spoke to me without the aid of an interpreter. He admitted freely that in the 1970s his company and others had perilously overfished Peru's waters. It was, he explained, the fault of the military government. No one really knew what was happening back then. No one thought about anchoveta biomass or fishing quotas.

But when we turned to omega-3s and health the conversation took a strange turn. He, like many of his generation, was worried about cardiovascular disease. He told me he'd had his blood tested and that his omega-6/omega-3 ratios were balanced. He had achieved this by sticking to a diet with lots of wild salmon.

Wild salmon?

I took a pause as I considered this. Here was the owner of the largest producer of *farmed* salmon feed in the world eschewing the result of his own product. Why? Because he felt that farmed salmon no longer had the omega-3 balance that he believed was critical for cardiovascular health. Salmon farmers had actually reduced the amount of omega-3-rich anchovies in their feed and gradually replaced it with omega-6-rich soy.

But what about the anchovies themselves? I asked him. Weren't *they* food? Didn't *they* have the right omega balance? What about the fact the vast majority of them were used for industrial purposes and not for human consumption? What about the fact that about 10 percent of the Peruvian population was starving and deficient in many of the nutrients anchoveta contained? Speziani agreed! Unsustainable! He even told me about a new product TASA was producing—something called the Omega Burger, a mixture of mashed-up anchovy thickened with squid and frozen into consumer-friendly patties. The Omega Burger, he explained, was one way TASA could gradually transform the anchoveta industry from reductionism to providing actual food for people. But, he explained, there were limits on what they could do. In the 1970s the Peruvian government had enacted a law requiring that nearly all the anchoveta catch *had* to be sold to the reduction industry instead of being used for human consumption. The law was the law.

"But wait a minute," I interrupted, "who wrote this law? I mean, presumably the industry, you guys, had some role in creating this law!" I said.

At this Speziani shrugged and smiled as he agreed.

"Of course, we are partially the culprits," he said. "We didn't see the future."

. . .

Not all of that anchoveta goes into fishmeal to be fed to salmon. The premium product today, once discarded or burned off because it soiled the meal, is the oil itself. Today it is distilled, encapsulated, and sold at a price that far exceeds what it might fetch if it was fed only to animals. The refining of this liquid gold was my final stop in Peru.

After my visit with Speziani, I dropped by TASA's latest project, a state-of-the-art supplement plant a few hours outside Lima. Prior to the construction of this plant, very little fish oil refining had gone on in Peru. Most of the raw material was spirited away, largely by Norwegians, and turned into capsules in the country that once burned herring oil for light. Now the Peruvians were reclaiming their treasure and refilling their rooms with gold. They had built their very own fish oil processing plant and were hoping to cash in on the ever-rising value of omega-3 supplements.

Compared with the fishmeal plant I'd visited earlier, the omega-3 plant was quiet and peopled by lab-coated scientists. Because omega-3s are extremely active, they can oxidize rapidly in heat. Many anchoveta boats lack refrigeration, so the product can degrade at sea. Chemical rearranging after harvest may occur to compensate. The ratios of EPA and DHA are adjusted, the triglycerides sometimes go through a chemical process called esterification. Nevertheless, inside the TASA lab, a Peruvian scientist named José Rainuzzo, who had trained in Norway and spoke of the natural gifts of the Peruvian anchoveta and advised taking a 500 milligram supplement daily.

"If I wanted to have the same effect by eating fish," I asked him, "how much fish do I have to eat?"

"Two anchovies," he told me. "Forty grams."

"If I eat two anchovies every single day, I am totally set for EPA and DHA?"

"Oh, yes, yes, yes."

But why all this? I wondered, as I took in the mass of infrastructure that lay spread across the plain.

Soon I was handed off to a towering Canadian named Dave Matthews. Just like the California reductionist Sal Ferrante before him, Matthews had been building plants all over the world, merging the activities of supplementism and reductionism. He seemed to like his work. He missed his children, his wife, Canada, and hockey—in roughly that order—but otherwise he was excited by the prospect of this plant, a node of supplementism in the very homeland of reductionism.

Matthews's big hand completely engulfed my own in welcome. He gave me a hard hat and steered me into a maze of pipes and ducts. He wore a confident, stalwart midwestern expression. When I told him that I had marginally high blood pressure he turned to the benefits of his product.

"So, you need to be eating two to three grams of omega-3 a day. . . . And that will take care of it. My cholesterol's extremely low, lower than my wife's, and she eats healthier than I do. And my blood pressure's extremely low."

I took in the scene, so completely different from anything

in North America, the wind howling across the plain, the Inca-faced descendants of Atahualpa busying themselves with forklifts and golf carts as they buzzed around the campus. Finally Matthews took me to the place where the oil itself could be viewed: a large metal bathysphere with a tiny window. I peered in and watched it slosh. It was slightly amber in color and ran clear as it whooshed up past the viewing window. It looked to my eye like a more viscous version of the colatura of the Amalfi Coast. But in this case all the deliciousness had been removed. The scent and flavor of the sea had been deconstructed into its chemical components and reassembled according to the requirements of the supplement industry.

What remained was an abstraction: medicine, not food.

Five

HEARTLAND

Supplementism and reductionism are sibling industries of a sort. They rely on the same animals and ecosystems to bring product to market. They also share an ideology to justify the boiling down of complex life into marketable molecules. In the case of supplementism, that boiling down is meant to address an imbalance in our bodies where an industrialized Western diet has removed many natural forms of omega-3s from our food. In the case of reductionism, it came about to address a dietary deficit in the diets of the animals we raise—an imbalance that occurred after we removed livestock from the ALA omega-3-rich grasses with which they evolved.

But over and above supplementism and reductionism, there is a much larger nutritional issue that modern societies keep circling but never really change: the overproduction of commodity-crop-centered foods that today can be found as readily in our school cafeterias as in our cupboards at home. These foods comprise the majority of our calories. They trend toward high amounts of refined carbohydrates, high levels of saturated fats, and, yes, low omega-3s and high omega-6s. A perusal of the top ten sources of calories in the American diet shows the general landscape:

1. Grain-based desserts (cakes, cookies, doughnuts, pies, crisps, cobblers, and granola bars)
2. Yeast breads
3. Chicken and chicken-mixed dishes
4. Soda, energy drinks, and sports drinks
5. Pizza
6. Alcoholic beverages
7. Pasta and pasta dishes
8. Mexican mixed dishes
9. Beef and beef-mixed dishes
10. Dairy desserts

The majority of these products are different expressions of three crops. The crop used to bring the meat-based products to market and create the sweeteners in those different desserts is corn. The lipid in all these high-calorie products is usually soy; 75 percent of the fat used in American processed food is soy, the second-largest commodity crop in the United States. Finally, the substrate used to make the more solid parts of all those cobblers and crumbles is wheat, 80 percent of these highly processed foods are so high in starch and sugar and so devoid of nutrients that, as the Mediterranean Diet scholar Walter Willett put it to me, "veterinarians would not feed it to their dogs."

A recent study in the *Journal of the American Medical Association* found that commodity crops could be linked to high body mass index, glucose-related abnormalities such as diabetes, and cholesterol imbalances. In summary, the study's authors concluded that "overall better alignment of agricultural and nutritional policies may potentially improve population health."

As of now, there is little sign of that realignment. Currently the federal government spends $15 billion annually propping up our current eating pattern. By comparison, Washington spends less than $1 billion on all fisheries programs combined. This persistent support of land food commodities translates into cost incentives that allow unhealthy eating patterns to persist. From 1985 to 2000, the cost of fruits and vegetables increased by 118 percent. During this same period the price of commodity fats and oils rose by only 35 percent.

The competition between nutrient-rich, omega-3-leaning foods and nutrient-poor, omega-6-leaning commodity foods can be described in two different ways, one chemical, the other systemic. The chemical argument posits that on a cellular level, enzymes that are the first step in metabolizing both omega-6s and omega-3s are, as the biochemist William Lands put it, "promiscuous and indiscriminate": they will work on an omega-6 just as easily as an omega-3, depending on what's most available. If there are a lot of 6s around, enzymes will favor them, which eventually produces compounds that are pro-inflammatory and linked to many Western diseases. If there are more 3s around, the enzymes will help produce compounds that slow the development of inflammatory compounds and lead to resolution.

The systemic argument, on the other hand, focuses on

high-calorie/nutrient-poor food versus low-calorie/nutrient-rich food. The oversupply of carbohydrates and empty calories a commodity-based diet provides leads to excessive weight gain, which in turn underlies many of the same Western diseases the chemical argument attributes to an omega-6/omega-3 imbalance.

Take, for example, type 2 diabetes. Diabetes occurs when the body loses its ability to process sugar. Type 2 diabetes is part of a metabolic syndrome that is strongly linked with obesity. Roughly 80 percent of those with type 2 diabetes are overweight. And if the American diet with its carbo-loading cakes and crumbles, its saturated beef and dairy, is anything, it's calorie intensive.

Omega World suggests type 2 diabetes may be ameliorated by correcting a deficiency in omega-3 fatty acids. Omega-3s could address type 2 diabetes by increasing "good" cholesterol, HDL, and decreasing triglycerides (two outcomes trials of omega-3s have shown, albeit with some inconsistency). But also, once again, inflammation is at the center of the justification for omega-3s as treatment for diabetes. "Obesity is associated with low-grade chronic inflammation characterized by inflamed adipose tissue with increased macrophage infiltration," writes Dr. Dyerberg in *The Missing Wellness Factors—EPA and DHA*. In other words, when a subject becomes obese, fat cells release chemical signals that trigger the immune system to come to their aid, as if they were being attacked by pathogens. This in turn creates inflammation. All this has led Dyerberg and others to conclude that "inflammation is now widely believed to be the key link between obesity and development of insulin resistance." Okay, sure. But what is the link between diet and obesity? Too many calories. And where are those calories coming from in the United States? Commodity crops. At the end of the day, it almost doesn't matter whose argument you choose. The dominant position of commodity crops in the modern food portfolio means that corn, soy, and processed wheat time and again win in the battle for money from our wallets and caloric space in our stomachs. Foods like seafood and leafy greens that are lower in fats and sugars and higher in omega-3s continually lose and cost more at the supermarket.

But what often goes unmentioned in the diagnosis of our food production disorder is an *environmental* competition that is being fought in the American heartland and in agricultural heartlands of countries around the world between commodity crop omega-6 systems and omega-3 systems. To get an idea of how the nation's native omega-3 system is being impaired by the commodities behemoth, it would be worth taking a summertime trip to the mouth of the Mississippi River, where most of the nation's fertilizer runoff exits into the sea. In certain places in the delta in July, if the air is still and hot, an event will occur that the residents of the Gulf Coast refer to as a "dead zone"—a blob of hypoxic water that has been forming in the Gulf since commodity crops started to boom in the 1980s. The Gulf dead zone has increased yearly to the point where in 2017 it exceeded eighty-seven hundred square miles, as big as the state of New Jersey. That this suffocation is taking place atop the most important commercial fishing grounds in the continental United States is indicative of this omega-3/omega-6 trade-off.

Dead zones begin when rivers carry nitrogen and phosphorus-based nutrients, primarily agricultural fertilizers, into the ocean. In the case of the Gulf of Mexico, it is the Mississippi River that delivers nitrates and phosphates from the American heartland into the Gulf at a rate of 1.7 million tons per year. Once this stew of nutrients reaches the ocean, algae bloom in prodigious amounts. When those algae die, bacteria consume them and draw oxygen out of the water in the process of respiration. In this way, bacteria suck the oxygen out of nearshore fishing grounds and suffocate the fish we like to eat.

The Gulf dead zone occurs far enough from shore that most people never get a chance to see it. But localized smaller dead zones (known on the coasts of Mississippi, Louisiana, and Alabama as jubilees) give an idea of what's going on. The bottom-dwelling flounder kicks things off. Sensing that there is no oxygen available, they will grow increasingly agitated as each successive gulp of water brings less and less refreshment across their gills. In a panic, the fish will head shoreward to the only breathable water they can find: the thinly oxygenated riffle the sea makes as it bumps lazily against the beach. At the shoreline, they will find humans waiting for them armed with "gigs," crude sticks with nails protruding from them. With an easy stab, each gigger will impale a suffocating fish, sometimes two at a time. Wading out farther, the fishermen will find sluggish pods of blue crab and brown shrimp. As the area slowly asphyxiates and the free-for-all reaches its climax, the human *whoops* coming from the darkness will give the impression of a happy time, a celebration of the ocean's seemingly endless gifts.

As industrial agriculture and animal feedlots have spread around the globe, dead zones have been spreading exponentially along with them. According to a 2008 study published in the journal *Science,* dead zones now affect ninety-five thousand square miles of water in four hundred different systems. They are as far-flung as the dozens of dead zones that have appeared off the coast of emerging Asia or as close to home as the Chesapeake Bay and Long Island Sound. But the place that tells the story of dead zones and the clash between seafood and land food is the Mississippi. A journey to those headwaters reveals the tensions contained within the river's twenty-five-hundred-mile journey to the sea.

The Mississippi River begins clear and cold at Minnesota's lovely Lake Itasca, a place where wild rice flutters in the shallows and remnant stands of old-growth oak and maple give a hint of what the world looked like two centuries ago, a time when millions of acres of riverside forest and hundreds of millions of acres of native prairie covered the Mississippi valley. But soon after the Mississippi exits Itasca State Park, the river begins picking up tributaries. The water turns a milk-chocolate brown. The forests fall away and are replaced by tilled fields. Along one of these tributaries I encountered the corn and soybean farmer Brian Hicks of Tracy, Minnesota.

Hicks is a kind and conscientious man who thinks a lot

about his farm and the impact it has on the surrounding environment. At the time of my visit, he tended to an orphaned deer on his property that ambled up and nuzzled me as I walked up his drive. He maintains stands of forest along the creeks that wend their way through his land, and his daughters are fond of pressing wildflowers they gather from the remnant patches of prairie that still dot the farm.

But along with his environmental responsibilities, Hicks has significant economic burdens. He is the father of ten children, and uppermost in his thinking is the agricultural machine that supports his family. "I tell lots of people that this farm is my factory," he said as we drove through his fifteen hundred acres that straddle the Cottonwood River, which feeds the Minnesota River, which in turn feeds the Mississippi. "Some factories make shoes. Mine makes corn and soybeans."

Hicks's Nettiewyynnt Farm has transitioned over the last 120 years from a diverse operation of livestock, vegetables, and grain to a business that focuses exclusively on chemically fertilized, genetically modified corn and soy. Today these are the number one and two crops in the United States. Together the American land planted in soy and corn would cover nearly two Californias. Much has already been written about the prominence of commodity crops in modern food systems. But what of the seascape and the food systems that existed before corn and soy took over the heartland? A look back to the time before the first pioneers reveals that water flowed quite differently.

"In Minnesota before settlers arrived we had eighteen million acres of wetlands," Jeff Strock, a professor at the University of Minnesota who works with Hicks on several agricultural experiments, told me. Those wetlands slowed the rate at which water entered the soil and allowed plants to take up excess nutrients before they hit the main stem of the river.

Which is why after farmers plowed the native prairie throughout the nineteenth and early twentieth centuries, they were forced to introduce artificially produced nitrogen fertilizers. Today, something like 30 percent of a farmer's annual budget is spent on fertilizer. And a huge amount of that fertilizer ends up in the Mississippi because of the way farmers have decided to deal with water.

Next time you fly over the Midwest, look down at the millions of acres of farmland planted in corn and soy below. Now imagine beneath all those acres a similarly expansive set of drainage tubes, funnels, and switches. This system is called tiling. Corn's growth rate slows when the soil is too moist, and farmers are forever at war with the environment to move water off their land. Tiling has been the principal weapon in that war. Today something like forty-eight million acres of American cropland have been tiled. In the Midwest, this extensive plumbing network often empties into tributaries of the Mississippi.

In some areas, farm runoff from tiling presents a major health risk. Since 2012, the city of Des Moines has been spending millions of dollars each summer so its utility can remove nitrate fertilizer from drinking water. Infants who drink water with nitrate levels as high as Des Moines' have suffered from something called blue baby syndrome, which can lead to asphyxiation. Medical reviews at the University of Iowa have also linked nitrates to cancer and immune deficiencies. All this makes citizens opposed to the behavior of large agriculture operations throw up their hands in frustration as they watch untreated farm water flow out of pipes into the municipal drinking water supply. "Look at the culverts discharging agricultural runoff into the Raccoon River"—the main source of drinking water for half a million people—says Des Moines Water Works utility manager Bill Stowe. "This is a publicly subsidized private plumbing system. They have the exact same configuration as if they were coming out of a city sewer." Unlike a city, though, agriculture has an exemption for storm-water discharge under the Clean Water Act. Stowe sued to block these upstream agricultural pollutants, but the closely watched suit was dismissed in federal court in March 2016. Nor is the Raccoon River and the greater Mississippi drainage the only place where this is occurring. A few hundred miles to the northeast, fertilizer-driven algae blooms spread out of the Maumee River in Ohio and for the last three years turned nearly a third of Lake Erie a sickening bright green, at times shutting down the city of Toledo's municipal water supply.

In spite of these increasing health concerns, the process of tiling and draining wetlands has only increased of late. And, again, it is the growth of a corn- and soy-driven food system that has put the pedal to the metal.

Perhaps the greatest cause of this acceleration is the shift of developing economies from native omega-3-based food systems to omega-6 ones. In China, beef consumption is trending sharply upward and is projected to nearly double in the period from 2010 to 2025. Along with this has been the same rise in poor health. The average Chinese citizen is now eight to fifteen kilograms heavier than the average a generation ago. With so many more Asians entering the middle class, they are moving away from a traditional diet of vegetables and seafood and eating more land food meat. Farmers in China and elsewhere in Asia have begun importing American corn and soy to feed their growing herds. True, Chinese use of American feed crops has slowed under the Trump administration, but in the face of the Trump tariffs, China has merely shifted its corn and soy needs to other countries like Brazil. And as of this writing, China had already begun to mend fences with the United States, desperate for even more corn and soy for its growing herds.

Corn prices have therefore trended consistently higher. By 2012, a China-driven spike put corn prices over 200 percent higher than a decade earlier. Prices have declined slightly since then, but the hope for another big boom means that the default is always corn. As you travel through the agro-industrial Midwest, you have the impression that the Mississippi River has faded from the consciousness of a region that once depended upon it. A river-oblivious industrial infrastructure has been overlaid on the American heartland, where a golden river of corn flows east and west by rail or truck, servicing the ever-growing demands of a world obsessed with corn-fed land meat.

This redirected flow of money has affected how farmers treat their land and correspondingly how they treat the Mississippi. As the beating heart at the center of the country's circulatory system, the river needs to process and balance all the runoff from all the surrounding land. Sometimes this runoff is natural—silt and soil that come off the mountains and plains in the natural process of erosion. But increasingly this runoff is coming off agricultural territory and is laced with many forms of nitrogen- and phosphorus-based fertilizer. And the territory the river drains is vast. Stretching from the Appalachian Mountains to the east and the Rockies to the west, it covers 1.1 million square miles—a third of the area of the continental United States.

Up until corn's recent price surge, a U.S. Department of Agriculture initiative called the Conservation Reserve Program (CRP) did a lot to keep dead zone–forming fertilizers from flowing into the Mississippi. Growing out of the post–Dust Bowl soil bank program of the 1950s, the CRP was officially established as part of the 1985 farm bill and paid farmers *not* to farm wetlands that are critical to fish. The price farmers were paid to refrain from farming these marginal lands usually bested what they could earn from planting them in corn. But today with foreign buyers competing for corn, crop prices are higher than any government conservation program can pay. Much of the land that was key to preventing nutrients from entering the Mississippi is now getting planted. A 2013 study in the *Proceedings of the National Academy of Sciences* revealed that from 2006 to 2011, farmers in the Dakotas, Minnesota, Nebraska, and Iowa plowed up 1.3 million acres of grassland and replaced it with corn and soybeans. That land-use change is of a similar magnitude as the deforestations taking place in the Amazon and is the fastest destruction of grasslands since the Great Plains were first plowed.

By the time I caught up with him, Brian Hicks was

desperately trying to find a compromise. His biggest attempt focused on the plumbing network that had been laid beneath his farm and that until recently was constantly sending fertilized runoff into the nearby river. As we cruised his fields in his four-by-four we came to a three-foot-high metal box that acts as a kind of switch to all the runoff that goes into the nearby river. While many farmers lack these control boxes and let their tiling flow continually, Hicks was proud to show me that he could time the opening and closing of his outflow, allowing water and fertilizers to be strategically retained in the soil and thereby not pollute the river.

He had other fixes. Back at his modest home tucked away in a copse of trees at the center of Nettiewyynnt Farm, he showed me his PowerPoint presentation with all of his stewardship ideas. Whether through GPS-based monitoring that allows him to pinpoint portions of his land that require less fertilizer or better tiling, or other ideas, it was in his interest to keep nutrients on his land because it makes his crops grow better.

"My feeling is that most farmers," he says, "they realize the dead zone is there, but I think they all feel like, 'You know, I'm one little farmer. . . . What I do can't really affect the Gulf of Mexico.' But what I'm reading and what I'm feeling and seeing is I know what we are doing as far as managing outflow is positively impacting the environment."

When you write about the environment, you always try to include stories like Hicks's. The drumbeat of the death of the natural world is deafening to readers, and the writer feels ever compelled to bait the hook, so to speak, with a solution around the bend. And when I met Hicks I sensed a heartfelt sincerity. No one wants to destroy his own backyard.

But still one could not help but notice that behind Hicks stood this edifice—this multimillion-dollar industrialized farm with reams of bills to pay that spoke to him in the grinding drone of corn.

And the more I looked into it the more I found food system thinkers who believe that everything farmers like Hicks are doing is nothing more than a Band-Aid on a gaping hemorrhage that started the moment settlers began their free-for-all on the prairie and sliced into the Midwest's native sod. In other words, the problem of nutrient loading into the Mississippi isn't the *methods* of commodity crop farming but commodity crop farming itself: an open-ended wasteful approach to land use that destroys the way that water, soil, vegetation, and nutrients reach equilibrium in a naturally composed ecosystem. Chief among those critics is Wes Jackson, until recently the director of the Land Institute in Salina, Kansas, and an oft-quoted spokesperson for the ending of farming as we know it.

"The essential problem is this," Jackson told me. "Humans went from perennial polyculture to annual monocultures. This in my view was the biblical fall."

Jackson's research has shown that the root structure of the perennial and diverse prairie grasses of the primeval Midwest extended more than a dozen feet down into the soil. When nutrients flowed toward the Mississippi and its tributaries they were intercepted by these root structures, processed, and dissipated. Indeed, Jackson's monitoring of a plot of prairie left in its native state on the Land Institute's grounds reveals that almost no nitrogen and phosphorus leave a field planted in native grasses.

This abandonment of native, deep-rooted grasslands that provided forage to grazers like bison and the early cattle in the United States also appears to have a health consequence that circles back to omega-3s. When animals are taken off grass and confined to stalls and fed primarily a diet of corn, they can suffer profoundly. In their natural state cattle live off a diet that leans in the direction of omega-3. Animals fed on grass ingest high amounts of plant-based ALA fatty acids, which they in turn can elongate into EPA and DHA. One reason is perhaps some of the farmers who transitioned from corn to pasture have found that their vet bills dropped markedly.

Indeed, when you look at how a grain-fed animal is twisted away from its grassland-based dietary norms and put on corn you literally see evolution turned against itself. Cattle have an organ called a rumen in which grass is fermented and broken down in a kind of predigestive process. A grazing animal typically has a neutral pH in its rumen. But as Michael Pollan noted in his *New York Times* feedlot beef investigation, corn causes the rumen to become acidic. Once this happens, animals have been known to go off their feed, chew dirt, paw at their undersides, and open sores in their hides. A corn-stuffed rumen can become overloaded with gas, producing far more methane than in a grass-fed animal. It is of course possible to mitigate the effects of a corn diet, and animal feed science has made significant strides since Pollan reported on the matter in

2002. As the animal welfare expert Temple Grandin told *The Washington Post* in 2015, "Grain is fine as long as there's plenty of roughage. . . . The problems come when you push too hard." Unfortunately the drive for cheaper and cheaper meat creates incentives for pushing hard, which can mean sicker cows and more methane. And methane as a greenhouse gas is ten times more potent than carbon dioxide.

In addition to chronic environmental damages like climate change, there are immediate health risks posed by CAFOs. Collectively livestock in the United States generate more than five hundred million tons of excrement every year, much of it coming from CAFOs. The waste gathers under industrial feeding barns and is eventually routed downhill to collecting ponds that the industry euphemistically calls lagoons. These stagnant stews of feces and urine pose a public health risk all on their own. True, some of it is used to fertilize crops, but there is far more of it than can be effectively spread on fields. Much of it lingers and in so doing pollutes the surrounding air with toxic chemicals like hydrogen sulfide and ammonia.

No one really cared about these sorts of things when the modern-day animal confinement system was created. What farmers transitioning from grass to corn noticed was the immense concentration of energy they could achieve by swapping grass with corn. But the large-scale replacement of prairie with row crops and CAFOs is just one aspect of land food's reworking of the country. A much more serious problem concerns the way agriculture has changed the very way that rivers flow—a direct and comprehensive reworking of the nation's very circulatory system.

. . .

Ninety percent of science is zeros."
    So proclaimed a spry, white-haired biologist out on an
expanse of big flat Mark Twain water near the city of Vicks-
burg, Mississippi. Paul Hartfield had just piloted a battered old
Fish and Wildlife Service skiff to a little eddy behind a snag of
old trees. With the boat secured he pulled in a wire mesh trap
baited with a can of cat food and found . . . nothing.

Hartfield had put out the trap the night before hoping to
catch samples of *Macrobrachium ohione,* a variety of shrimp that
lives in the Mississippi. Before my visit with Hartfield I'd
always thought of shrimp as saltwater creatures, catchable in
edible quantities only in the near- and offshore waters of the
world's oceans. But ten years earlier Hartfield had stumbled
upon the river shrimp. And when I came to know this oddly
overlooked creature, I came to understand what was happening
to the Mississippi delta and the incredible wealth of seafood
that it supports.

Hartfield's life is one that has been governed by the flow of
the Mississippi and the creatures that inhabit it. After serving
in Vietnam in the 1970s, he returned home, where he took a
job with the Mississippi Museum of Natural Science in Jackson. In 1979 a biblical rain swept up from the Gulf and caused
the adjoining Pearl River to burst its banks. Water sloshed into
downtown Jackson and inundated the museum, playing havoc
with the archives of shelled creatures stored in the museum's
darkest corners. Particularly ravaged was the collection of
freshwater mussels. Though not a mussel biologist by training,

Hartfield had a knack for general taxonomy; he spent months identifying and relabeling the collection. It was thanks to these frequent visits with the storm-buffeted mussel collection that he reacquainted himself with another biologist he had known in high school and who was now the museum's science director. Several months later, Libby and Paul Hartfield were married. Their bond to this day is built upon a shared appreciation of the river that flows near their door.

From that point forward, Hartfield embarked on an unusual scientific career—unusual in that it defied the narrow row most biologists find themselves hoeing for the length of their careers. In his biological journey he crossed over from creature to creature, from taxa to taxa, to come to know the ecosystem of the lower Mississippi in its entirety. He helped secure endangered species status for the Alabama sturgeon. He helped popularize the eating of invasive Asian carp. He has identified countless bird nesting sites in the old cottonwoods that dot the floodplain. But it was the river shrimp that helped him pull together many different threads of thought and determine what the river and all the seafood we derive from it had suffered.

River shrimp, Hartfield learned, had in precolonial times not just made a quick jaunt from the lower river to spawn in the sea; in fact, some juvenile shrimp swam upstream into the upper reaches of the Mississippi's main eastern tributary, the Ohio River. The mature females eventually returned to the estuary, completing a round trip of more than three thousand miles. And because they made such an epic journey and interacted with so many human population centers they were a major source of food. In 1899, two hundred thousand pounds of river shrimp were taken by the commercial fishery of the Mississippi, and we can assume many more, perhaps orders of magnitude more, were caught and never reported.

In the present era, when he took me out on the river we found only one or two shrimp per trap. Where had they all gone?

The natural way of the Mississippi (and indeed all rivers) is to wend and flood. The turning of the earth bends a river askew from the gravitational pull downhill. Eventually the river corrects itself and starts heading down again, only to be bent once again by the spinning earth. The result is a flow of water that twists one way, then another all the way from the top of the country in Minnesota to the bottom in southern Louisiana. In addition, most rivers in their natural states flood and expand to many times the width of the narrow channel we associate with inland watercourses. The combination of a slow winding course and a wide floodplain meant that the river in its unmodified state allowed plenty of time for suspended nutrients to drop out of the water column and fertilize both the river bottom and the surrounding plains. Indeed, it was this wide floodplain that made the Mississippi valley the fertile treasure so many farmers coveted. In addition, the nutrients that settled into the riverbed provided an ample base for organisms at the bottom of the food web. This in turn encouraged higher and larger forms of life to prosper. Based on what fisherman catch in the river today, some might think Twain's Huck Finn a liar for claiming to have caught a two-hundred-pound catfish from the Mississippi. A look at the way the primeval river worked, though, backs ol' Huck up. Even the river's very name seems to say so. Though the generally accepted Indian meaning of the name Mississippi is "Father of Waters," some etymologists believe the name stems from the language of the Outouba tribe in which the word *Missi* meant "everywhere" and *sipy* meant "river." "The River That Is Everywhere" is a much more apt description of the way the river worked when it was free of the tinkering of humans—a sloppy mess of a basin where water does what it wants to do.

But a river that is everywhere, a river that follows its own vagaries, is hard to colonize. The untamed Mississippi overflowed its banks every year, and in certain years the river up and moved completely. Channels that were one year navigable by steamships the next became dry sandbars. In response to one cataclysmic event—the Great Flood of 1927, the greatest inundation the United States had seen in its short history—farmers of the young nation decided: enough. The river had to be contained.

"The Army Corps of Engineers wanted the river to be faster and shorter," Hartfield told me as we hauled anchor and sped farther upriver to find more shrimp traps. "Most engineers said it was a bad idea. They knew even back then that the river has a way of finding its own equilibrium. But they did it anyway."

Over the course of the next three decades the Corps cut off the river's oxbows and deepened its channels. The Mississippi was shortened by more than 150 miles. In some places the Corps raised the entire river high above the floodplain. Locals refer to the Mississippi at these points as a "perched river," a river you literally have to look up at, flowing above, bound up in straight-jacketing sets of levees. In this way engineers spurred on by farmers transformed the greatest watercourse in the continental United States from a big, easy, diverse, fish-productive system to a more sterile straight shot to the Gulf of Mexico. The sediments that once dropped out and fertilized the country all up and down its length are now carried along in the radically swifter current and spirited into ocean waters off Louisiana. There all of that nitrogen-rich water does nobody any good. In fact, it does harm. The nutrients that would have normally settled out and fertilized the floodplain instead fertilize the ocean, annually enlarging the Gulf dead zone and contributing to marsh loss along the coast. It is, in fact, a kind of devil's bargain, a gradual elimination of a seafood system in favor of a land food system. River shrimp that once fed on the settled out nutrients in the river and then eased upstream in slow, manageable currents to spawn in the headwaters are now blasted downstream and limited in their ability to spawn and forage.

It's worth noting that these kinds of land-food-for-seafood trade-offs are as old as the settlement of the Americas. Long before they invaded the Mississippi valley, European immigrants transformed the natural way that rivers and seafood systems work throughout the original thirteen colonies. In early New England, local governments subsidized the construction of dams in nearly every major watercourse—dams that blocked and eliminated stupendous runs of salmon, sturgeon, shad, herring, and other omega-3-rich fish. The town of Dedham, Massachusetts, granted one Alexander Shawe sixty acres of land in 1637 in exchange for building a corn mill. In 1680 the

town of Andover, Massachusetts, offered free timber and real
estate to any citizen who would put up a gristmill on the Shaw-
sheen River. New Englanders answered the call for more dams
with full knowledge of the damage they were inflicting on migratory fish. By the modern era dams were everywhere and fish
were nowhere. Every one of the more than four thousand dots
on the contemporary map of my home state of Connecticut
below is a dam.

In spite of what is in effect a national, subsidized campaign
against rivers, Paul Hartfield believes there are small fixes we
can make to reverse some of the damage. Heading west from
Jackson, across the broad muddy river, he spoke about his long-
standing negotiations with the Army Corps of Engineers.
"The Corps are focused on what's out here," he said, indicating
the main part of the river where government engineers try to
maintain a safe and efficient navigable channel. Up ahead, we

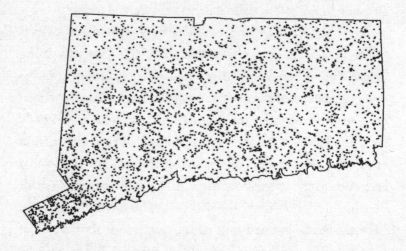

came to a turnoff, and he veered his skiff off to the left. "Me, I'm focused on what's in here."

In a little while, we turned into a different habitat called a backswamp—an eerie forest of half-submerged trees. A pair of green-and-red navigation buoys and other random refuse, which had been flushed from upstream, bobbed by. "This is a peaceful spot to contemplate the dissolution of the elements," Hartfield mused.

Hartfield envisions a series of minor changes using the model of this quiet little patch of backswamp. He has been trying to persuade the Corps to create modest redirections of current that do not affect navigation but at the same time move more water into floodplain channels and swamps. "These small local modifications," he said, "can be constructed during routine maintenance and construction activities at no extra cost to the taxpayer."

The swamp's impact on water quality is immediately visible. On the upstream side of the backswamp, several miles away, the water entering the floodplain was a milk-chocolaty brown, rife with all the sediments and nutrients that farmers had put into the river far upstream. As we emerged on the downstream side, water flowed out of the vegetation almost translucent with the deep green color of living algae luxuriating in a liquid feast.

"All the leaves and stems of the vegetation growing in the swamp slow that water down, and the sediment drops out," Hartfield said. "When the water clears and sunlight gets in, the algae bloom and consume the nitrogen and phosphorus in the water. Really, when you think about it, a floodplain is a river's kidney."

After our day out on the river we retired to the solid pine, cypress, and ash house Hartfield had built with his own nine fingers. (One finger was lost when, rushing to complete his previous hand-built house twenty-five years earlier in advance of his daughter's birth, he switched from hand tools to a radial arm saw and promptly cut off four of his fingers. A friend scooped up three of them, and they were successfully reattached.) There, after our meal of wild catfish, a storm brewed. Lightning flashed all around. And then the largest thunder crashes I had ever heard blasted in the heavens.

"Don't worry," Hartfield said. "After my last house burned down, I totally overbuilt this one." On and on through the night the storm raged. The old house shook and rattled. All the power that the wind had built up rushing across the Great Plains slammed into the dwelling. The rooms were illuminated by so many lightning strikes that it seemed like dawn. It was a night that was to become known in the South as the night of a hundred tornadoes. The next day, as I drove downriver toward the Gulf, I listened to the car radio describing how all up and down the length of the Mississippi the river was rising. In some areas of the Midwest, levees had blown out and water was rushing to inundate acres upon acres of corn and soy.

The river was everywhere.

Severe floods in the heartland seem to be intensifying year by year, and during particularly intense storms, the runoff of fertilizers into the Gulf of Mexico swells. The dead zone grows in lockstep. Spring 2017's epic inundations were to result in the largest Gulf dead zone in recorded history, so large that researchers who track its size never reached its western end.

As I watched reports of the dead zone coming in, showing the red blob of hypoxic water spreading daily—the result of a torrent of fertilizer flooding down into nearshore waters of the Gulf of Mexico, choking out the shrimp and red drum, the blue crab and flounder that could have provided so many healthy meals—I couldn't help but think of what Hartfield had told me when I asked him what he'd do if he could have all the money he wanted and could reengineer everything in his path to bring back the Mississippi River shrimp and help all the other creatures that live in the greatest fishery in the continental United States.

"If I had all the money in the world?" he said, considering the big flat open river before him. "I'd move the levees back five miles, then turn it all into a park from Cairo to Baton Rouge. Then I'd leave it alone and let the river fix itself."

If we were to measure the overall value of a seafood-friendly, less commodity-intensive diet, we might perhaps take seriously some of the more radical propositions for reforming the heartland. A wider floodplain, more native grasslands, healthier grazing animals, and a more seafood-rich Gulf of Mexico would likely translate into significant savings in health costs. Perhaps a food economy based on seafood, grass-fed animals, and leafy greens might even bring greater economic benefit to the country. But there is one other large force at work in America's heartland that short-circuits the bigger dreamers' dreams.

That is the simple fact that large portions of the American agricultural system are not devoted to food at all. Today around 40 percent of the corn produced in the American heartland is used to make automobile fuel. From 2001 to 2010, ethanol production grew by 700 percent. This growth, once again, is driven largely by subsidies.

"Do we produce a product that is good?" Brian Kletscher of Highwater Ethanol asked me in his office as rows of trucks loaded with corn rumbled past the window into his refinery. "We do. I think we've got it right. The U.S. farmer has been able to make some dollars this year."

But while the U.S. farmer may have been able to make some dollars, the overall equation is not always favorable. A review of a host of studies presented to the U.S. Congress on ethanol production found that at best a gallon of fuel has to be burned to get 1.5 gallons of corn ethanol. Some studies determined a net energy loss. The average seems to be that a gallon of gas will get you about 1.2 gallons of ethanol. Not a very promising ratio. The industry argues that it has grown ever more efficient, so that the burning of oil to produce still more oil works out in the end, at least for the farmer. But one can't help looking at this giant edifice of activity as so large that it follows its own logic, irrespective of whether it serves the higher logic of the planet.

Interestingly, though, there is a way of addressing the agricultural/energy overlap that again loops back to a more omega-3-friendly way of doing business with the planet. This was something I encountered in the last leg of my journey through the American heartland, in the sizzling west Texas town of Midland.

"I always tell people when they come to Midland," the algae farmer Isaac Berzin said as he welcomed me to George W. Bush's hometown, "I always say, 'This is a reminder to be good in this life. Because this is what hell feels like.'"

Heat rose in wavy filaments from the roadbed. And as if to remind you that fossil-fuel-driven climate change was behind a good portion of that heat, oil wells were everywhere. Next to playgrounds, alongside strip malls, in school parking lots, in private owners' backyards, like those dipping birds one sees at curio shops, dipping and dipping into the ground, pulling up more and more crude, helping make Midland 112 degrees in the shade on a July afternoon. Never before have I seen the cause and effect of climate change so closely juxtaposed.

That Berzin would greet me with a suggestion to be good or face the consequences of hell was very much in keeping with his interesting blend of moral and scientific education. He had originally set out to be a philosopher at Ben-Gurion University of the Negev in Israel, but after he overheard a discussion among a group of engineering students, he approached the head of a nascent biotechnology department and changed his major. He wanted to *do* something, to change something. For him, that something quickly became algae.

"Look, the original plan," he told me as we shot down the arrow-straight road toward Imperial, Texas, "was not to make omega-3s. Not at all. What we wanted to make was jet fuel." This is not such a crazy idea when you consider where our

modern-day petroleum comes from. Ultimately most petroleum is fossilized algae. Indeed, when Berzin ran his *Nannochloropsis* algae ("nanno," as he lovingly calls it) through a gas
chromatograph, he immediately saw two large spikes on the
carbon graph for C16:0 and C16:1. The very carbon chains
that are the stuff of high-energy fuel.

By 2006, Berzin's trials showed the potential to generate an
economically credible amount of fuel from an algae farm. He
even got grants from the U.S. Department of Energy to move
the project forward. But eventually the project crashed and
burned. A global petroleum glut had just hit the world, and
suddenly oil had fallen to below $60 a barrel. Algal oil, while a
genius and ultimately sustainable idea, could not survive in the
economic environment of subsidized ethanol and full-bore petroleum exploration.

Berzin returned to Israel, took a good job at a private university, watched as his daughters went into the Israeli army,
and prepared for something of a semiretirement.

"But, you know, I couldn't do it. It was like those two people who talk while the soccer match is going on."

"You mean the commentators?"

"Yes, yes. I was a commentator. I wasn't a player. I knew
there was something there." But what?

What Berzin really wanted to make was a new kind of fuel
that would help the world avoid the worst ravages of global
warming. But what he realized was he would have to find a
more viable economic hook on which to hang his algae idea. It
was then that he returned to the gas chromatographs and considered what else algae had to offer. The offerings turned out

to be considerable. Along with the peak for the C16 molecules he wanted to burn as jet fuel, there was a second peak even higher for C20:5. When he looked into those peaks he realized they represented the presence of molecules that had a high commercial value; in fact, they were the same peaks that Jørn Dyerberg had observed all those years ago when he'd drawn the blood of seal-eating Greenland Inuits: EPA and DHA omega-3 fatty acids.

Berzin set out to learn more. He read about all the effort and potential environmental disruption that was being caused by mining the oceans for them. And he realized it just might all be totally unnecessary. He happened to recall a key story from his university days about the discovery and production of the diphtheria vaccine. When diphtheria was first isolated in the early twentieth century, the medium that was used for incubating the vaccine was the blood of live horses. Initial plans for mass production of the vaccine required the killing of thousands, perhaps hundreds of thousands, of animals. Eventually, though, an artificial pathway was found and the vaccine was cultivated in the laboratory. The "middleman" of the horse, as Berzin called it, was cut out entirely. The vaccine became cheap, efficient, and widely available, and millions of lives were saved.

What if, Berzin wondered, you could do the same with omega-3 fatty acids—cut out the middleman? Remove the Peruvian anchoveta and Chesapeake Bay menhaden from the whole process? What if you could go right to the source of the very organisms that made omega-3s, the very creatures at the bottom?

Berzin's narrative converged with our arrival at the algae farm itself. Located just off the highway was a small encampment of aluminum trailers adjacent to covered sluices of green water.

"Isn't it kind of not so environmentally friendly to be pumping water here in the middle of the desert?" I asked him.

"Ah," he said. "Let's not ruin the surprise."

Leading me to a hydraulic lift, Berzin strapped me and himself into harnesses, pushed a button, and raised us high above the algae farm.

"You asked me earlier about water," he said as we dangled in the glare of the hundred-degree heat. "That was my challenge when I started this project. I wanted to grow something that took no arable land and no freshwater. All of this water here is brackish."

It turns out that the land we were surveying was land already wrung dry by modern American land food agriculture. In the nineteenth and early twentieth centuries much of it had been in corn and cotton and the aquifer beneath it had been ruined. As is happening to aquifers all over the United States, and indeed all over the world, the water had turned uselessly salty from too much irrigation. Aquifers can be drained only so much before the prevailing mineral profile of the surrounding land taints them. For human nutrition it was now a dead zone. Nothing could grow there. Nothing, that is, except algae.

Because the types of algae Berzin had selected can tolerate a wide range of salinity, the brackish aquifer was perfect for them. Moreover, because it comes from underground sources, the water can be seeded with a culture of the particular EPA-rich strain of algae Berzin prefers without being infected by competing algae.

I asked Berzin the usual questions I'd asked all the proponents of omega-3s about the controversy surrounding its demonstrable versus its proposed human benefits. He shoved over a paper on depression and said unenthusiastically that this study offered considerable proof on omega-3s' efficacy against it. But to my surprise, when I pressed him for other studies he gave up and shrugged.

"Let me ask you this," I said. "Do you take omega-3 supplements?"

Here Berzin lowered his head and smiled abashedly. "I really should, you know. I have marginally high cholesterol."

"But you don't?" I asked.

"No, I don't. My daughter's in medical school. She's always harassing me about it."

"But do you really believe in omega-3s?"

Here Berzin considered the moment carefully. He inhaled and rolled his eyes as if trying to remember all the various studies he had read as to why this formulation of EPA and DHA prevented heart disease or why that phospholipid was particularly bioavailable. But all at once he exhaled and seemed to visibly drop his pretenses.

"There's something else, isn't there?" I asked.

"Yes, of course there is!" he said, throwing off the supplement talk like an old skin. "These algae are 40 percent protein!"

"So?"

He pushed the button on the crane, dropped us down to earth, and rushed me into one of his trailers. There he put on a PowerPoint presentation, brought up a slide, and toggled me through the ten-thousand-year expanse of human agriculture and animal husbandry. "First you have cattle. Five hundred acres and four hundred tons of carbon to bring a kilogram to the plate. Now look at pigs, a little better, but still, not very good. Now here's chicken, still lots of acres, lots of land needed, lots of water. Soybeans, not much better than chicken. Kind of surprising, right?

"Now, look here. Look at the algae. One acre produces almost ten thousand tons of protein per year. With a soybean you have to grow an entire plant with leaves and stems, etcetera, to get this one seed. With algae you use the whole thing. The oil goes into the omega-3 supplement. The protein goes into artificial meat products. And that's it."

He told me that it was important to remain focused. That he'd been through enough business cycles to understand that when you lost focus you lost your business. And right now what he was focusing on was the supplement business and omega-3s. A kilogram of algae used for fuel brought in about fifty cents. The same kilogram for protein, between $8 and $15. A kilogram for supplements? Bingo—$20 to $40. It's not that he didn't like the idea of supplements; it's just that he was reversing the old equation that the Romans had done with garum and the Peruvians had done with anchoveta. He was using the co-product, supplements, as a means for exploring a whole new food and energy economy. He understood that his was an early step. But at the end of the day a person's got to make a buck.

"So you're saying it could be a kind of . . . food?"

"Yes. I'm saying Texas, the place that produces this long-horn cattle, this beef that Americans love, that this is not the right thing for this land now. Believe me. I am from Israel. Israel I like to call the canary-in-the-coal-mine country. All of the things the world is about to experience—heat, lack of freshwater, food insecurity—it already hit Israel. And I'm telling you that *this*—this, my nanno, this thing, is the only solution that we have."

"And if petroleum ever gets any more expensive?"

"If oil gets more expensive, we can beat them too. Who needs oil wells when you have nanno?"

The sun had arced lower in the sky, dissipating the heat ever so slightly and suggesting that it was time to shoot back down the arrow-straight highway from Imperial to Midland to catch my evening flight. We sped away from the algae farm, on toward town with oil wells pumping on either side of us. We passed the occasional herd of beef cattle that had only now ventured out from beneath the few isolated shade trees. Both of them, the cows and the oil wells, seemed, in the beam of Isaac Berzin's bright intellect, shadows of an increasingly out-of-date way of thinking—fossils of another era that he and his omega-3-rich algae could someday make entirely irrelevant.

Six

AT THE BOTTOM
OF IT ALL

The chinstrap penguin crossed in front of me and stopped cold in his tracks. He seemed to be weighing, on the one hand, the idea of getting his mouth around all the omega-3-rich krill that had gathered at the green edge of an iceberg near shore and, on the other, the possibility of a seal getting its mouth around his own oily body and biting him in two. He glanced over at a pair of penguin feet that had been shorn from their owner by just such an encounter. He took in the hundreds of krill-tinted vomit piles and the acres of penguin droppings that brought a particular penguin-ish stench of fish, feces, and oil to the air. He looked up at the crowded penguin colony on the hill, forty thousand pairs, each braying and fighting over nesting pebbles. That prospect seemed equally unappealing.

So the chinstrap penguin stayed where he was. And I did too. Even though the last call had been made for the landing craft to return to my mother ship, I waited. I had to.

In Antarctica the penguin always goes first.

When you decide to write a book profiling a single thing—a fish, a philosophy, a color, or, God help you, a molecule—you inevitably head off on tangents that seem to take you far from your original subject, from algae, to colatura, to ethanol, to, well, penguins. The author Michael Pollan, who had bumped up against omega-3s in his research for his book *In Defense of Food*, warned me at the outset of my fatty acid project that it would be hard to retain focus. "Once you start down this tunnel," Pollan wrote "it explains everything—like Causabon's Key to All Mythologies in *Middlemarch*."

But there is one very far-flung tangent that eventually circles back to the very heart of the matter: climate change. Both climate change and omega-3s hail from the same source: the carbon bonds contained within the membranes of photosynthetic phytoplankton. Some of those bonds ended up in petroleum, others were expressed as long-chain EPA and DHA fatty acids. Whether we incorporate them into our cell membranes or burn them in the flume of a power plant is a matter of evolutionary chance and contemporary choice.

Looking at this convergence helps us grasp the degree to which we are turning the power of the ocean against itself. Destruction of the world's fish-producing rivers and the propagation of dead zones is acutely affecting natural seafood-producing systems around the world. The reduction industry's removal of forage fish from their critical place in marine food webs resonates throughout the waters off the shores of every continent. But the human reworking of the chemistry of the entire ocean dwarfs all other problems. Time and again the ocean has bailed us out at moments of near extirpation. It is still bailing us out in the form of a carbon sink. To date the ocean has stored a major portion of the anthropogenic carbon we've put into the atmosphere since the Industrial Revolution.

But as we continue to burn billions upon billions of fossilized phytoplankton, rereleasing ever more carbon those organisms sequestered so many millions of years ago, we may have at last exceeded the ocean's ability to compensate for our bad behavior. Land-based food systems are a major contributor to this problem, from the methane expulsions of our cows to the acres and acres of forests felled to make way for lowland soy production to the billions of gallons burned to drive land food agricultural equipment. And even though it's many thousands of miles from the American Midwest, Antarctica, that wildest continent of all, may suffer the most devastating effects of a human food system that has turned the land against the sea.

The trip across the Drake Passage from Argentina to Antarctica was unusually calm. A "Drake Lake," as one of the scientists joked, instead of the sixty-foot swells that sometimes rage across its depths. The calm weather afforded me the chance to peruse maps and understand a bit more about where I was headed. About halfway through my crossing, time became profoundly unimportant. As I sat in my tiny cabin looking at the different charts and maps on the walls, one in particular struck me. It was a map of Antarctica in which the time zones had been delineated more or less in line with each country's claim to sovereignty.

It was one of the most absurd maps I'd ever seen. There is not much reason to have time zones or even time for that matter in Antarctica—all the world's longitude lines converge there, and for much of the year the human conception of day and night is not particularly relevant. Though many nations have tried, no one has come to possess Antarctica. The time zones shown on the map were a suggestion that should the place one day get divvied up, time should be apportioned along lines of foreign sovereignty.

For me, the only way I could mark time was to close my porthole, which I did one "evening," only to wake eight hours later, open the porthole, and see a series of icescapes radiating such a supernatural, cerulean blue that it made me feel as if I had passed through the wardrobe into Narnia. Within a few hours of my wandering about the ship trying to figure out which portion of it connected with which, a call came out, old as the Antarctic/human relationship itself: "Whale!"

Ahead was not the sad spectacle of whale watching I'd experienced in the past, when a lonely cetacean beat a circle around a dismal tin boat off Cape Cod. Here was what the Norwegian captain Carl Anton Larsen saw in 1903. It was this kind of abundance that drove him to cajole Norwegian financiers into sinking millions of kroner into a fleet of ships that would transform the largest animals the world has ever seen into sticks of margarine. Now whale spout after spout filled the air with mist. Here and there flew pink plumes of krill— orange, lipid-rich, full of the antioxidant astaxanthin that in the endless polar day acts as a kind of planktonic sunscreen.

Flexing their tails with their caudal peduncles, the strongest muscle in the animal kingdom, the whales moved foot by foot, up, up, up, slowly, almost like the slow strobing of a rocket just barely achieving liftoff from its silo. Then, as if the launch were aborted, they slid just as smoothly and slowly back into the water with no sign of disaster below other than the ring of krill they left in their wake.

Since the whaling moratorium went into effect in the mid-1980s, the great whales have been spared, save those that are still killed for a largely politically motivated research program conducted by the Japanese. Slowly whale numbers are beginning to build. No longer are the giant factory whale ships from Norway hounding them. As cold and harsh and windblown as the environment felt as I peered over the side of the ship, it was also oddly peaceful. Just a family group of whales sitting down to eat krill in the long single day of the polar summer.

But then I noticed, off the port side, a vessel not here to look at whales: it was a krill boat, here to harvest what the whales were eating.

On the bridge I found the captain, a Swede named Leif Skog, charting a course through the ice-strewn islands that surround the Antarctic Peninsula. Skog checked the myriad instruments on his panel and identified the boat as the Norwegian vessel *Saga Sea*. Skog had seen it working the same area on the previous month's cruise.

"First they're gonna clean this area out," Skog said, "then they're gonna go clean somewhere else." On another monitor with sonar readings he showed me an electronic haze on the screen that extended downward. "That's about thirty meters deep. Maybe a ship's length across. All filled up with krill."

In the last ten years krill has become the omega-3 industry's new darling child. It represents the largest single-species animal biomass in all the world's oceans. Actually nobody really quite knows how much krill there is down at the bottom of it all. Estimates range from 300 million to 500 million metric tons. By comparison, the weight of *all* the fish humans take from the sea annually is 80 to 120 million metric tons. The contemporary krill catch is modest in relation to its estimated population—around 200,000 metric tons. One hundred sixty thousand metric tons of that catch is caught up by a single Norwegian company called Aker BioMarine. The company is rightly proud of its methods. It uses a patented vacuum tube process that literally sucks the krill out of the water without sucking in anything else. When I later visited Aker's "krill logistics hub" in Uruguay, it was as if I had come upon some Dr. Seussian vision of a newfound thneed. Sacks and sacks of pink krill dust were piled high to the rafters of the warehouse en route to a krill oil refinery in Houston. When packaged and inserted into ruby-red gelcaps it is the most expensive supplement of all, often retailing for more than $40 a bottle.

But here off the Antarctic Peninsula, it wasn't a supplement. It was whale food. What's more, a naturalist along on the trip told me, many of the whales feeding were pregnant mothers.

That krill would now be a target of the very same nation that had removed a large portion of the Southern Ocean's whales seemed more than ironic. But to point fingers only at the Norwegians is to miss a larger truth of the White Continent. Antarctica is both a real place and a metaphor. It marks the outermost boundary of the manifest destiny fantasies inherent to seagoing nations. Throughout the last phase of Southern Ocean whaling in the 1940s and '50s, the Soviet Union, Japan, and the United Kingdom all aspired to make a piece of Antarctica their own. Cold War paranoias were invading the thinking around the continent at the time and there was a justifiable fear that this last wild place would succumb to the same sorts of divisions that were fracturing the world into communist and capitalist spheres of influence.

The language surrounding Southern Ocean whaling reflected the bellicose nature of the times. In 1952 the vice-captain-director of the Soviet whaling vessel *Sovetskaya Ukraina* told his crew that they "should leave a desert behind us." The Soviets very nearly did, removing 180,000 more whales than they reported to the International Whaling Commission. The same behavior was witnessed in other Soviet Antarctic fisheries. In an illicit letter to Greenpeace written during the Gorbachev years, a Soviet fisheries inspector named Oleg Senetsky railed against his native country, "whose main task is to catch more and more tonnes of fish paying little attention to national and international regulations. Deep concern for the condition of the Antarctic ecological system (as for any other), for the idea of turning Antarctic into an international nature reserve made me to look for any possibilities to express my views to any influential persons or organisations beyond the borders of my country."

When the global whaling moratorium was put in place, the Soviets redirected their Antarctic fishing effort toward krill. By the 1980s, Soviet vessels were taking more than half a million metric tons annually. But just as the out-of-control Soviet whaling industry was, as one Soviet historian put it, a reflection of "the U.S.S.R.'s desire to do everything bigger and better than other nations, especially those in the capitalist world," so too were plans for krill expansive and not altogether logical. No one can say for sure at this remove what exactly the Soviets were up to with all that krill. It is possible that a certain imperial pretension prompted them to want to keep an economic placeholder in the White Continent. The UN Convention on the Law of the Sea had just come into effect, extending national zones of influence out to two hundred nautical miles. This forced Soviet fleets out of the territorial waters of most nations. Antarctica was still open for fishing, and it made a certain global chess player's sense to move parts of the fleet into those icy waters. It's also possible that the whole venture was a giant make-work scheme commensurate with the larger Soviet agenda to achieve maximal employment for the proletariat. One anecdote that circulates among Antarctic scientists is that the Soviets were stockpiling krill as a protein source in the event of a global thermonuclear war. Soviets also reportedly tried feeding it to livestock. Just as menhaden and anchoveta were useful for pig nutrition, the Soviet scientists reasoned, krill could feed an army of chickens and put a chicken in every Soviet pot. There was one flaw in this plan. Because krill contain large amounts of fluoride in their shells, they become toxic to nonmarine animals. A sliver of evidence in the academic record also suggests they tried feeding it to mink. Fur, at the time, was an important Soviet export, tradeable for desperately needed hard currency. Perhaps krill gave sable a more lustrous pelt?

But in investigating the Soviet Antarctic adventure, one also finds more hopeful examples of human behavior. The reason why Antarctica is a place where wildlife is largely recovering rather than spiraling downward is that the very urges of mutual destruction that fueled the Cold War reached a point of stalemate on the White Continent.

In 1957, in the wake of Joseph Stalin's death, after years of mutual paranoia, an international clutch of scientists managed to convince their governments to launch what was to be the greatest sharing of scientific information in the modern era. The so-called International Geophysical Year was timed to occur during a period of maximum solar activity—a time when scientists hoped to collaborate across enemy lines to maximize what could potentially be a year for groundbreaking observations. It was also a year that followed humanity's entry into space and the first reckoning with the fact that nations were merely passing manifestations on a planet that was now visually documented as a shared home. In this brief window of rationality, the Soviet Union and the United States and all the parties active in Antarctica realized that no one could afford to expand the Cold War's frontiers to include this last cold patch of land and sea. The best and safest way to avoid hostilities on the White Continent was not to issue any claim at all.

When, much later, in 1982, signatory nations to the Commission for the Conservation of Antarctic Marine Living

Resources (CCAMLR) wrote a founding charter, they lay a groundwork, unique in the world, in which the default principle was to leave life alone rather than exploit it. Today in Antarctica, with the significant exceptions of krill and a few species of fish, you simply cannot disturb wildlife in any way. If a penguin crosses your path in Antarctica, you must not interfere with its crossing. It is because of the underlying philosophy of conserving rather than exploiting life that today in the Antarctic, the penguin always goes first.

Reflecting on this legacy, as I looked off to port and saw the *Saga Sea* patiently working a suction tube into a mass of krill, I felt a mix of emotions. I knew that relative to the total biomass of five hundred million metric tons, the annual Norwegian take of less than two hundred thousand tons of krill was quite small. I knew that the vessel was deploying a recently invented device called an Eco-Harvester that kills almost no other creatures besides the targeted krill.

But I also knew that a fight for Antarctica was going on clear across on the other side of the Southern Ocean in the Tasmanian city of Hobart. There, CCAMLR signatories were debating whether to create the largest marine reserve in the world, a 598,000-square-mile area in Antarctica's Ross Sea, twice the size of Texas, 70 percent of which would be completely off-limits to fishing. I also knew that signatories to CCAMLR had allowed a "rational use" clause to be inserted into the CCAMLR founding documents, leaving the Antarctic door open to future exploitation. And I knew that the world's emerging krill barons just might contest the Ross Sea reserve because, who knows, what if such a restriction was extended to the waters of the Antarctic Peninsula, the most krill-laden waters of all?

The work aboard the *Saga Sea* carried on. Somewhere on board, the crew had readied a tank of cold saltwater. Because krill store their oil in a space between their muscle tissue and their carapaces, they must be handled gently if the oil is to be secured for its high-end markets back in the Northern Hemisphere. Old school Soviet trawlers trying to spirit their hundreds of thousands of tons of krill back to Russia in the 1980s often ended up crushing their quarry, leaving vast plumes of wasted oil bubbling in their wakes. The Soviet krill exploitation scheme was also foiled by the fact that krill have highly active enzymes and immediately begin digesting themselves upon death, turning their crisp inch-long prawn bodies into orange-pink goo. Now that Norwegians were trying to sell krill as a premium product and not just as animal feed they were much gentler with it. The suction hoses and the cooling tanks they used kept the little blobs of pink oil beneath the krill's carapaces intact and stable for transport.

China had designs on using a similar operation. Even as it emulates the Western diet with more and more grain-fed meat, it is similarly emulating our supplementation pattern. China is now the fastest-growing market for omega-3 supplements. Perhaps because of that trend, the chairman of the China National Agricultural Development Group recently declared in a press release, "Krill provides very good quality protein that can be processed into food and medicine. The Antarctic is a treasure house for all human beings, and China should go there and share." China has asserted that it has a right to raise its krill harvest to two million tons, arguing that this would still leave hundreds of millions of tons to feed the marine life of the Antarctic.

Looking at the estimates of current krill populations, it does indeed seem like there's a lot out there. But when we imagine Antarctica as a blue-ice heaven, among the most unspoiled places in the world, we have to remember that it is still only a remnant of its former purity and abundance. No human had ever set foot on the White Continent until the American sealer John Davis stepped upon the ice in 1820. A decade later most of Antarctica's large seal colonies had been savaged. When humans first developed boats fast enough for whale hunting and flotation devices to suspend the carcasses of the great whales so that they wouldn't sink to the bottom after harpooning, there were many hundreds of thousands of blue whales. Now there are just a few thousand. Before the advent of whaling, penguins ate a much more diverse diet simply because there was not as much krill around as there is today. The whales were eating it all. Whereas krill once represented only 25 percent of the Gentoo penguin diet, today it is 70 percent of their nourishment. Clearly, the presence of whales in historic numbers would require much, much more krill. So when we talk about leaving enough krill for wildlife, are we talking about leaving enough for what we have or what we'd like to get back? A vision of the past or of the future?

Much more important are far more sweeping changes to the ocean—changes that are particularly apparent in the Antarctic.

Ecologists typically describe Antarctica as a "wasp waist" ecosystem with krill acting as the narrow pinch point in the middle. Below that waist sit countless species of phytoplankton, which share a common predator: krill. Above the krill wasp waist swim penguins, seals, whales, a host of fish, and albatross that wander thousands of miles to scoop up their oily goodness. Unlike ecosystems to the north, which might have other prey to dilute the effort of predators—squid, small fishes, crustaceans of various kinds—in the Antarctic only krill have the right metabolic tools to survive the extremes of light and cold. They are alone in their ecological niche.

This is partly to do with the way that krill have figured out how to endure a night that lasts 180 days. Krill are phytoplankton-dependent, and bloom following a phytoplankton bloom. When the first light of the Antarctic summer dawns in late October the water is crystal clear. But by the time full summer comes on in February what was once clear, lifeless water turns a murky green—a field of phytoplankton, ripe and fatty—just the thing that krill like to eat. As I cruised around in a Zodiac one afternoon, I could see the phytoplankton starting to build to their summer numbers. The bases of the icebergs were tinted green, ripe for harvest.

In an era of climate change, however, the water is warming and the warmer environment seems to be selecting for smaller species of plankton. If this trend continues it could interfere with the growth and abundance of krill. Later, when I brought a krill back to the laboratory and looked at it under a microscope, I could see a basket of tiny "feeding" legs the animal uses to ensnare long chains of diatomic phytoplankton and gobble them down. In the warm summer months, krill prefer gorging on the blooms of larger diatoms. But it was recently found that a low amount of winter sea ice produces a smaller amount of winter phytoplankton followed by a smaller summer phytoplankton bloom that produces more small species and fewer large ones. This means fewer large, juicy diatoms for the krill.

And this sort of disconnect could happen throughout the seas. A warmer ocean is likely to be an environment that selects for smaller phytoplankton. If that was to happen we could see the gradual emergence of something called a microbial loop. In such a scenario, smaller phytoplankton, which have shorter life spans, never get a chance to feed bigger, more complex animals. Instead, they fall prey to bacteria and exit the food chain as fodder for microbes. The result is a downward spiral—less complex systems that feed microbes rather than fish, penguins, and marine mammals.

There is yet one more krill/phytoplankton interaction that is changing. In a place like Peru, the cycle of diatoms ebbs and flows as the days shorten and lengthen. In the Antarctic, there is a complete shutdown of photosynthesis when winter arrives. How then do krill survive? The key is in the ice itself. As sea ice starts to form, it entraps strands of diatoms, putting the organisms into a state of suspended animation. Small droplets of these phytoplankton cling to the underside of the ice, and as juvenile krill rise in the water column to forage in the long Antarctic night, they scrape the bottom of the ice with their tiny mandibles, eking out a tenuous existence.

Sea ice serves an additional function. When spring finally

comes in November, the algae trapped in the ice act as an "in-oculation," infecting the surrounding water with a culture of active cells. The water warms, the sun rises higher, the algae divide, divide again, and again and again. The cycle of life is renewed in full force.

All well and good. A brilliant adaptation to a difficult problem.

But what do you do when the blackness of winter still comes on schedule in March, but no ice forms?

B ob Jacobel, a glaciologist from St. Olaf College who had accompanied me to Antarctica, tried his best not to put his nose into the krill mess. Like any good scientist, he is loath to extrapolate beyond his area of expertise; that would be conjecture, not science. Bob's area is ice. Over the course of many years, he worked on the Antarctic ice, missing a dozen Christmases while deep in the field. Laughingly, he recalled now how in the early years he'd phone in his Christmas wishes to his daughter, Allison, via the ham radio operators:

> *Hi sweetie, this is Daddy: over*
> *Merry Christmas, Daddy: over*
> *Merry Christmas to you too: over*
> *I love you, Daddy: over*
> *I love you too, sweetheart: over*

Allison had dreamed of joining her father on the ice someday, saying when people had asked about her father's whereabouts during those lonely Christmases of the 1990s that "Daddy was busy at the bottom of the world." Now on this particular trip, at twenty-eight, Allison was finally able to come down to the bottom with him. She had just finished a PhD at Columbia University analyzing diatoms in ocean sediment for evidence of climate change. On the fourth day of the voyage, the three of us were thrown together into a Zodiac, and we skimmed along the edge of a glacier and talked about the geologic cycles that were now affecting krill and indeed all of planetary life.

Around us were astounding shapes of ice glowing with an otherworldy blue. It was as if some manically productive sculptor-giant was constantly whittling out divinely inspired creations, holding them briefly in a palm, and then tossing them over the shoulder to begin working on another dozen masterpieces. Some of these masterpieces were huge. In Antarctica, one is always having to adjust for scale. Ahead was a wall of ice that seemed at first like the buildings in my neighborhood in Manhattan's financial district. But when I took into account our distance from the ice wall I realized the scape before me was as big as the entire territory of greater New York City, all of it apparently stopped in time like a portrait. But, Bob explained, the appearance of motionlessness was an illusion.

"You can see up there, it looks just like a river," he said. "If you had a super-speeded-up camera you would see that it has rapids and slow bits, even eddies of ice spinning around. But we don't, so maybe that's why some people don't believe what we're saying." To the west of us, the ice shelves that surround this part of Antarctica are beginning to give way. They currently act like a cork, keeping the West Antarctic Ice Sheet in place. With the shelf ice now melting and calving into the sea, the West Antarctic is starting to move. Its eventual collapse is now considered inevitable. When it falls into the water, seas all over the world will rise about 10 feet. Should the much larger East Antarctic Ice Sheet eventually go, Jacobel says, the rise will be more than 150 feet.

That the observed changes in west Antarctica would be occurring so fast seemed to strike Bob in a strange way, as if his very past were being erased before his eyes. He had been coming down to the Antarctic on and off for over three decades. His career had overlapped with the step-by-step discoveries that led us to realize humans are playing an active role in changing the earth. Some of those trips were to do geophysical scouting, looking for places that would be suitable to drill ice cores—miles-long cross sections of ice that would later be taken apart, centimeter by centimeter, and analyzed to reveal the exact composition of the atmosphere when that ice was formed. For many seasons Bob scouted, taking a series of flights first from New Zealand to McMurdo, the largest American base in the Antarctic, indeed the largest human settlement on the entire continent with the staggering population of twelve hundred souls during the summer research season. From there, he would fly to a deep field camp hours away from that already remote base. He and sometimes as few as three other scientists would camp out to complete their surveys.

Sometimes flights out would be delayed for days or weeks. Once, when their team had completed its work and a plane approached, the scientists joyously dumped their stove fuel and water to make sure the loading would go more quickly. The pilot, not liking the landing conditions, banked and turned away and ended up not returning for several days. The scientists were left to scamper around the camp area, collecting canned fruit and any unfrozen liquids. When I asked how he could possibly have borne this and returned year after year, Bob looked at me wide-eyed with disbelief at the silliness of my question: "It was the science!"

Bob was helping to prove that the world's climate changed in synch with carbon. Among the early formers of this hypothesis was a scientist named Milutin Milanković, who showed that the great planets of the solar system affect the earth's orbit ever so slightly, changing its tilt and orientation in relation to the sun in very regular ways. These slight changes alter the amount of solar radiation reaching the poles and bring on ice ages and warm periods in between. Once Bob and others started analyzing ice cores, they found that the quantity of carbon dioxide in the ice cores matched both the air temperature and global ice volume almost exactly, and that the periods of these variations fit the pattern of earth's orbital changes. CO_2 built up as temperature increased and ice melted, and declined when the temperature dropped and an ice age began. A graph of the carbon levels in the samples showed a pattern similar to a human pulse, but with tens of thousands of years between heartbeats.

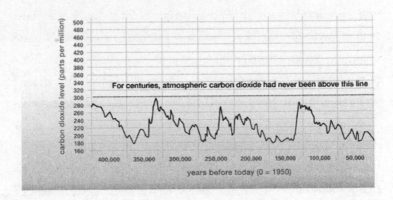

The predictability of carbon rising and falling in a cyclical pattern seems reassuring. It seems to say it might get hot or cold, but all of it is part of a larger cycle. But if you move the graph forward to the year 1950, the reassuring pattern falls away.

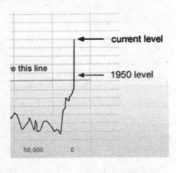

Carbon shoots up completely out of alignment. For the first time in observable geologic history, the atmospheric carbon cycle is out of synch with Milanković's wobble.

And so is the temperature. In a sense, we are doing more to change the earth than are the pull of Jupiter, Saturn, and the sun combined.

I can hear the voices of climate change denialists screaming in my ears. If I am inferring causation from the observations made by this host of different scientists, aren't I making the same claim that Omega World makes when it associates high omega-3 levels with myriad positive health outcomes? Two factors persuade me that the case for human-caused climate change is much stronger. First, you cannot design a randomized controlled trial for the earth. There is no second earth that you can add carbon to at will to see if there's an effect. With scientific problems of this magnitude we can only do what doctors would call retrospective association studies. Yet there have been so many different kinds of association studies in so many fields of earth science that find the same correlation between carbon and climate that to me, causation is the most statistically valid conclusion we can reach.

Second, we know that temperature, carbon dioxide, and ice volume are closely linked through the ocean, the atmosphere, and all of the earth's living organisms. The climate system is driven by the orbital variations on long timescales and those variations are reflected in every measurable system we have discovered to date. True, the geologic record does not show the effects of an abrupt increase in CO_2 such as the experiment we are now performing. But the physics of adding greenhouse gases to the atmosphere are very straightforward and well understood. Add CO_2 and the temperature goes up. That fits very well both with our model of the past and with what we are observing today.

What human-driven climate change means for krill is that its habitat is changing quickly and dramatically and will soon differ radically from the habitat with which it evolved. While climate change skeptics are quick to point out that there is just as much, if not more, sea ice today in the Antarctic than was present a decade ago, nowadays the period when the sea is covered with ice is noticeably shorter, especially in places that tend to have much larger aggregations of krill. In 2016, sea ice reached its maximum much earlier than average and declined rapidly thereafter, leading to a new record sea ice low for the month of November—a million square kilometers below the previous November. This sets up a potentially disastrous situation for both krill and their forage. Previously, when the summer light faded, photosynthetic algae started to die. But they were saved from complete extirpation by being frozen into sea ice. If no sea ice forms before the light goes away, this suspended animation trick doesn't work. And in spring when the sea ice melts, there will be less and less algae to start a new culture and to feed juvenile krill.

So when supplement companies speak of an epic supply of krill available to both whale and human, they may not be taking into account the full effect of the change to come. In some areas, particularly around the Antarctic Peninsula, krill populations have declined by as much as 80 percent in the last forty years. Should the climate continue to warm and the sea ice form even later, that loss will surely become more severe. Some studies have suggested that as much as 80 percent of the present krill habitat will be gone by 2100.

There was to be no Drake Lake on the passage home. Already as we pulled away from the last finger of the Antarctic Peninsula, the beginnings of a significant storm caused the vessel to take on a heavy roll. I sat in the library trying to ignore the anxiety I felt about where we were headed—both literally and figuratively. In times when disaster feels close at hand, I often take comfort in some other distant distress. Any ripping yarn of daring survival will do. Now I paged through the accounts of Antarctic explorers of days gone by who had endured much more difficult trials. Douglas Mawson, who trekked for days through a blizzard across the Antarctic plain and was forced to strap the detached soles of his own feet back on with twine—only to watch from a bluff while his rescue vessel sailed back to Argentina, leaving him to spend a second consecutive winter in the dark. Otto Nordenskjöld, who on learning that his ship was trapped in winter ice ordered his men to kill and stack 280 penguins for both food and fuel (a penguin is so thoroughly soaked in krill oil that it burns like a Duraflame log). Roald Amundsen, who had beaten Robert Scott to the South Pole by committing the ungentlemanly atrocity of "pyramiding" his dogs—that is, designing his expedition with the gruesome intent of feeding sled dogs to sled dogs to fuel the trip home.

When I tired of these grisly tales I turned to the ship's science library and read about still more terrifying things forthcoming, even if their horror could be grasped only through the lens of a microscope. Driven by an overproduction of carbon dioxide, the global ocean is acidifying at a faster rate than at any other time in the last fifty-six million years; calciferous phytoplankton may be starting to dissolve in that acidity. A controversial recent study found that the standing stock of chlorophyll has declined in over 62 percent of the global ocean surface area—some of the largest declines occurring where I now sailed in the Southern Ocean. Whether this is due to warmer waters and more zooplankton predators, or to a change in ocean chemistry, we can't yet say. The trend is disturbing, regardless of the cause. Meanwhile, due to increasing turbulence driven by the rising intensity of storms like the one that was now buffeting my ship, there was a chance that something the science writer Alanna Mitchell referred to as a "methane burp" might escape the deep ocean and enter the atmosphere. For millions of years methane gas that is formed by decomposing organic matter in the ocean's lowest depths has been kept sealed in by cooler ocean waters. But as waters warm, the ceiling on this methane hell house could come off. As a greenhouse gas, methane makes carbon dioxide seem like child's play. Should this ancient methane bubble belch out, it would tip the world's climate toward something so inhospitable that all debates about omega-3 or omega-6 would seem triflingly irrelevant.

But as I steadied myself against the ship's roll, I tried to think about what we could throw up in defense against the gloom. And here Antarctica was itself such a shining example: the only continent in the world where the international community had jointly decided not to fight a war over territory. A place the world had universally decided to share. A place where the International Geophysical Year was celebrated like a Christmas of Christmases and where the gifts exchanged were the highest scientific findings swapped freely among a hundred nations, hostile and friendly alike. A place where the murder of half a million intelligent creatures was largely halted and mourned. Where an ozone hole is being gradually plugged by the soundness of an international accord supported by some of the best science the world has ever seen. What was most important was the Antarctic commitment to complex ecosystems. Antarctica's scientists had said no to mineral extraction, petroleum extraction, and even, to a large degree, single-species reductionism. We were only now starting to see the dividends of that effort.

Just as our vessel was hitting the highest of seas in the middle of the Drake Passage, the signatories to CCAMLR were preparing to come to the table for their next meeting. Atop the agenda was the designation of the largest marine reserve in the world. Nearly six hundred thousand square miles in the Ross Sea. Over the course of the last ten years, one by one, a number of nations had warmed to the idea. The last holdout had been Russia. Its scientists, the "technical intelligentsia" as they're known in that nation with one of the greatest scientific traditions in the world, were slowly convincing their politicians of the supreme rationality of it. Eventually the Russians would come to terms. The marine reserve would be created. "The room just erupted," one observer of the meeting in Hobart later told me. "We had a sense that we had done something incredibly significant." As of this writing the protection of the Ross Sea, the largest marine reserve in the world, is law. Throughout large swaths of this new reserve, everything is protected. Even krill.

Out the window, the storm raged. Thirty-foot swells crashed against my little porthole. Pressure waves of spray made the hull shudder. Staggering out to the rear deck, I breathed in the last air of Antarctica as we crossed the "Roaring Forties"—that howling block of latitude that separates the White Continent from the domesticated world to the north. As I clenched the rail choking back a particular combination of nausea and nostalgia for a place that I probably would never see again, I leaned my head back and saw a dark shape hover over me and then drift back toward the boat's wake. It was one last bit of wildlife that I had been hoping for during the trip but not yet seen: an albatross. On the passage out, with only minimal wind, these largest of seabirds with wingspans in excess of twelve feet couldn't get enough lift to fly. A Drake Lake is no place for the emperor of all gliders. Now as the winds moaned a fifty-knot dirge and whipped the sea into a mad foaming torrent, the great birds took flight and slipped over the whitecaps, their steady gazes calm and cool, as if lofting along with a light summer breeze.

Seven

TOWARD AN OMEGA-3 WORLD

When I started out on my investigation of omega-3s, I had wanted to find a way of eating that was good for me and good for the planet. I had hoped that the omega-3 could lead me to that solution. It did, but not quite in the way I expected.

After four-odd years of staring at this strange little family of molecules, there is only one conclusion that seems to match their potential: their power lies in their tendency to indicate health more than in their ability to cure our ills. Quite simply, omega-3s are the molecules of coolness and wildness, of wellness and a balanced diversity. Their elimination from our food system reflects their elimination from our world. The planet gets hotter and simpler with every new phase of human expansion, while humans themselves drift toward chronic illness.

Driving factors for this decline of health and diversity are the shallow-rooted commodity crops that largely determine how we eat today. It is these crops that displaced the perennial grasslands which once sequestered carbon and stabilized aquatic environments. It is with these crops that we turned grazing animals away from their natural fodder and transformed them into factories for fat and protein. It is this commodity crop system and the associated concentrated animal feeding industry that together generate the second-greatest amount of CO_2 after power production, and more methane and nitrous oxide than any other anthropogenic source. It is this system that takes our three principal macronutrients—carbohydrates, fat, and protein down a winding road away from nutritional and environmental balance.

Let's start with carbohydrates. In the United States, corn occupies the lion's share of our arable land, ninety million acres, roughly the size of the state of California. Corn grown year after year depletes soil fertility. To prop up that fertility, we first raided the sea. We turned to forage fish like menhaden and Peruvian anchoveta for fertilizer, which in turn diminished the availability of nutrients to larger, more palatable fish. When fish became too expensive to simply bury in the ground, we turned to chemical fertilizers and used fish as a supplement to perpetuate concentrated animal feeding operations. Chemical fertilizers and animal feedlots overenrich estuaries and cause harmful algal blooms and dead zones, killing still more fish. All in the service of producing carbohydrates, which some dietary studies suggest are overrepresented in the Western diet.

When it comes to fat, again contemporary land food production leads us down an unhealthy path away from the omega-3s. Much of our cooking oil and around three-quarters of processed food products contain omega-6-rich soy, a crop that expanded in the American heartland through the draining of swampy, marginal areas. These wetland ecosystems are critical to the propagation of juvenile fish and shellfish. By removing those areas and converting them into soy farms, we have cut off our nutritional nose to spite our face. And as with corn, soy less and less goes to feeding humans. Most of it goes to feeding land-based livestock in concentrated animal feeding operations, one of the largest generators of greenhouse gases in the world.

Perhaps the most upsetting part of this trend is that a large portion of the feedlot meat that is causing so much ecological damage is actually far in excess of our nutritional needs. This brings us to the third leg in the modern dietary stool: protein. If there is a macronutrient of the moment, surely protein is it. Protein is promoted everywhere: in whey-based supplements, in energy bars, on breakfast cereal packaging. But when you dig into dietary recommendations, it turns out that our need for protein is actually relatively small. The U.S. Department of Agriculture recommends that a typical male consume around 90 grams of protein a day and a woman around 60 grams to maintain a lean body mass.

What does that translate to in terms of actual food? Ninety grams of protein is the equivalent of one thin McDonald's hamburger a day, a little more than half of that for women. Unlike carbohydrates, which we convert to fat in times of plenty and use later in times of paucity, protein can't be stored in great quantities by the human body. Indeed, one of the reasons why high-protein diets have become so popular is that we can eat a lot of protein, fill our stomachs, and never have to pay the price in weight gain later on. The human body simply excretes whatever protein it cannot use.

This reality is hardly mentioned when food companies and associated scientists warn us of an impending "protein deficit." The standard line at conferences on food production and sustainability is that we will need to double protein production in the next fifty years if we are to accommodate an anticipated population of nine billion humans. Dig down into the numbers and another story emerges. Nearly half of that new protein production we "need" is not to meet the recommended daily allowance of a larger population. Rather, it is based on shifting the lower-protein dietary patterns in developing nations to the protein-oversaturated patterns of developed nations. Just as the people of Crete in the early Mediterranean Diet studies *wanted* more meat but didn't need it, so too do people in poorer countries want more animal flesh, probably because they perceive it as a symbol of progress. They want, in other words, what might make them sick.

Before the developing world heads down this aberrant road we must resist wants and urges and look at what the Mediterranean Diet really teaches us: that a diet with minimal amounts of animal protein and saturated fat and high amounts of fruits and vegetables is about as healthy a diet as humans can muster. The question then presents itself: how do we get more people to accept that truth? Perhaps that motivation could come from where it always has: the selfish human desire to live longer.

. . .

Steve Gaines is a marine ecologist at the University of California at Santa Barbara who, during an earlier phase of his career, was instrumental in designing marine protected areas—underwater reserves where fishing is severely restricted or banned outright. He was a key scientist in advising the closing of 16 percent of California's marine waters to fishing and the subsequent creation of the United States' largest network of underwater reserves. His goal had always been to try to get the word out about the fragility of marine wildlife. A fish kept alive in the water was, for Steve Gaines, a positive in the balance sheet for the planet.

But when he became dean of UCSB's Bren School of Environmental Science & Management in 2010, he was tasked with looking beyond his earlier fish-saving mission. In so doing, he started to wrap his head around which large-scale changes in human behavior would do the most to limit humanity's damage to the planet. The most realistic change, Gaines realized, was food.

Food, he came to understand, accounts for a major portion of resource use: 70 percent of the earth's freshwater, 30 percent of the world's energy, and 36 percent of the planet's arable land. When he considered these large numbers he began discussions with a renowned ecologist named Dave Tilman who had begun a visiting professorship at UCSB. Tilman was also trying to understand the impact of the 50 percent increase in human protein demand many researchers predicted would occur by 2050. Tilman had assessed the impacts of such an increase using land-based sources of food only and concluded, as Gaines relates, that "they were all bad options." But as Gaines pointed out to Tilman, there was a major source of protein that had been left out of his analyses: the ocean.

Gaines had already been doing some back-of-the-envelope calculations on what would happen if we rebuilt every over-fished wild fishery and returned it to stable productivity. At most, he concluded, rebuilt wild fisheries would likely contribute only about 5 percent more food to humanity's growing demand. But when Gaines started looking at aquaculture the results were "consistently better and in many cases dramatically better than anything we had on land." This was true across all four metrics of resource use—fossil fuel consumption, freshwater, land/ocean conversion, and nutrient loading. It was also true across a range of behaviors by farmers. Even a very average grower of seafood had fewer environmental impacts than most land food meat producers.

Even more compelling was what Gaines found when he started looking at his results relative to a large-scale meta-analysis Dave Tilman had just completed on the health effects of different diets. In 2014, Tilman published a paper in *Nature* in which he examined the life spans of subjects observing vegetarian, pescatarian, and Mediterranean diets versus a conventional Western-style diet. Surprisingly, vegetarian diets performed similarly to the conventional diet in terms of all-cause mortality. But both Mediterranean and pescatarian diets showed a 15 to 20 percent increase in longevity.

When Gaines and Tilman began analyzing these studies to solve for the best combination of low environmental impact and strong human longevity, the results strongly favored a pescatarian-oriented diet. In other words, a diet that had as its root animal protein, seafood, particularly what Gaines calls "non-fed" aquacultured protein: mussels, kelp, and a whole range of other bivalves and marine vegetables that draw their nutrition from the sea and sun alone. One might call it the Pesca-terranean Diet.

How, then, do we get to a point where the Pesca-terranean Diet is the norm rather than the exception? How do we escape the land-centered industrial food monolith we have manufactured for ourselves?

Some might take the solution I'm driving at to be a complete abandonment of terrestrial agriculture. But before the reader bolts for the seafood counter, it's important to note that a Pesca-terranean Diet is not an all-fish diet. Not at all. In fact, as part of the research for this book, I tried to see what would happen if I turned to the sea for the bulk of my calories. For thirteen months, I replaced land animal meats with seafood, much of which fell into the oily, high-omega-3 category. During that time I ate over forty pounds of wild and farmed salmon, twenty pounds of anchovies, ten pounds of mussels, and a random other thirty pounds comprised of mackerel, sardines, summer flounder, halibut, lobster, shrimp, tuna, striped bass, and bluefish. But when I sat down with my general practitioner and did a before-and-after comparison of the standard markers that are used to make risk assessments for cardiovascular health—cholesterol, triglycerides, blood pressure, heart rate—my doctor could detect no change.

While it's possible that these standard markers of Western

medicine might improve over a longer trial period, and while it's also possible that the benefits of an all-seafood diet might be measured in more abstract terms (a longer life, for example), the problems of complete pescatarianism are manifold for other reasons. My mercury levels as measured in hair samples more than doubled during my trial period. PCB concentration probably also increased.

No, what I am suggesting is *balance* built along Mediterranean Diet lines but with a greater inclination toward the sea. Remember, in all forms of the Mediterranean Diet, a limiting of *all* animal protein—marine and terrestrial—is key. My proposal is that we aim to restrict ourselves to a very modest animal protein component in our diets and that we should consider omega-3-leaning animal protein as the source for that very modest component.

How might we go about this in a global way? To my mind, it is a little bit like balancing the arms of a scale. Currently, industrial land food has tipped the scale so far that we are perilously in danger of falling flat on our faces. What we need to do is ever so slowly add weight to the ocean side to lift the burden off the land and bring the system into equilibrium.

Easing the weight on the land side of the scale will require our rethinking and rebuilding terrestrial food systems in a pretty major way. To do so we will need to try to emulate the endemic ecologies we destroyed when we implemented large-scale commodity crop and feedlot animal production. As of this writing such a solution is nearing realization in the Kansas town of Salina. For the last twenty years, Wes Jackson, the agronomist who had first introduced me to the vital role native grasslands had played in precolonial America, has been trying to recreate those same grasslands in a way that can be useful to humans.

The key to this attempt is a perennial grain crop Jackson's team has been developing called *Thinopyrum intermedium*. It has only now just entered market as Kernza—"kern" from kernel and "za" from the end of *Konza*, the Native American word from which "Kansas" was derived. Whereas annual crops like corn and wheat are planted and torn up every year, Jackson's perennial Kernza stays in place, allowing humans to harvest its seeds again and again without disturbing the soil. In such a system, soils are stabilized and industrial fertilizer is greatly reduced; the loading of nutrients into watersheds is similarly diminished. In addition, the extensive root system of Kernza also manages to store a lot more carbon than do corn or soy. In precolonial days, midwestern grasslands had extensive root systems, sometimes a dozen feet deep. The world's primeval grasslands were carbon sinks rivaling the oceans in their ability to take CO_2 from the atmosphere and literally bury it in the ground. Kernza performs the same function while also providing edible grain. And so, conceivably, if Kernza was developed as a keystone crop, it could transform the modern farmlands of the Great Plains from carbon leakers into carbon reservoirs.

Of course, the kinds of seeds that would be produced from a Jacksonian agricultural system would be of a different nature than the ones currently grown. Unlike corn and soy crops, which go into industrial products like ethanol, high-fructose corn syrup, and cattle feed, Jackson's crops would primarily feed people. Instead of a commodity-based agriculture system that sacrifices the health of adjoining water bodies, Jackson has proposed a flipping of the system. "If you take our 328 million acres of cropland, right now it's 80 percent in annuals and 20 percent in perennials," he told me. "My proposal is that at the end of fifty years, we would have 20 percent annuals and 80 percent perennials.

"We can do it," he continued, "but it will take a commitment from our society to get that done. This is what the U.S. Department of Agriculture should be working on instead of accommodating the cattle and pig welfare program." Jackson is something of an outlier in the world of agriculture, and his program has yet to turn a profit. But keep in mind that the corn and soy agricultural complex is supported by $15 billion in farm subsidies. If even a small portion of those funds could go toward developing alternative, sustainable grains, very slowly the behemoth supertanker of industrial agriculture could start to tack away from its destructive path toward a more constructive future.

That said, there is a problem with Kernza. Yield per acre is about 25 percent of the total energy calories produced by wheat. But here is where the nongrain portion of the plant kicks in. In addition to its seed crop, Kernza produces abundant leaves and stems that make excellent cattle feed. The Land Institute's plant breeder Lee DeHaan wrote me from Kansas that the leafy green portion of the plant is as high in protein and energy as most planted pasture, particularly if it is grazed in the springtime. "In the big picture," DeHaan wrote, Kernza "is a pasture grass, so most general statements and findings about the feeding of cool-season pasture grasses will apply to Kernza residue also." In other words, it will likely have a fatty acid profile like most cool-weather grasses—imbued with decent amounts of ALA omega-3 that grazing animals can elongate into EPA and DHA. There is even some initial evidence that pasturing animals on Kernza extends the seed-bearing life of the plant, making it all the more productive.

The grazing element of Kernza brings me to the second major omega-3-driven reform of land food that would substantially change our ecological impact as well as our nutrition: a transition from grain-fed, feedlot animal husbandry to a kind of enhanced pasturing system.

If you were looking for an example of someone who has been through all the conflicts between commodity crops and natural systems and come out the other side in a better place, Guy Choiniere in Highgate Center, Vermont, would be it. Choiniere is a fourth-generation Vermont dairy farmer. His certified organic operation sits on 450 acres of rolling land that today embodies the romantic ideal of the well-managed farm. A little over a decade ago, though, Choiniere's farm was muddy and manure-laden and a direct threat to Vermont's whitefish, trout, and salmon in nearby Lake Champlain.

"There wasn't a blade of grass on those riverbanks," he told me as we ambled over native clover and vetch. "The cows were destroying it. There were landslides every other year. Conservation is about keeping your soil and your minerals on your own farm. And that's exactly what I wasn't doing. I attracted attention long before these rules were mandated."

When soil conservation inspectors first started snooping around his property in the late 1990s it was hard to take. "Someone coming onto your farm and telling you you've got problems is very insulting," Choiniere recalled. "We had to get over that." Ten years later, it was clear he was very much over it. Now beneath his barn were catchments that slowed drain water and caused it to percolate slowly through the soil, filtering out nutrients. Leading down to the river was a lush forest that had been planted with the most efficient trees for uptaking nitrogen and phosphorous before it could hit the river and cause an algae bloom.

Eventually Choiniere made a leap of faith and went a step further. He ripped up his cornfields and planted his land back into native pasture. Since pasture is never tilled, it holds the soil much better than does an annual crop like corn. There are other benefits. His ruminants are eating what their rumens were built for: fermenting and digesting grass. The omega-3 health benefit they receive from the evolutionarily correct elongation of short-chain fatty acids into long-chain results in much healthier animals. Ever since he went to grass-fed, Choiniere's vet bills have plummeted from $15,000 a year to $500. The price he earns from his milk has risen 15 percent and he spends no money on tilling.

"Being sustainable is money in my pocket," he told me as he looked over his fields of green. "That's the name of the game for staying in business. Agribusiness will give you recommendations all day long. How much fertilizer to use. How much grain to feed. . . . Me, I went with my instincts."

It is easy to imagine a future in which Choiniere's fields planted with Wes Jackson's Kernza might prove both sustainable and profitable. Such a system would be based fundamentally on the power of omega-3 and could better protect both nearby watersheds and the fish they contain.

There's one more switch land food producers could make that could improve soil and water quality while at the same time maintaining a healthy economic environment—a switch from farming corn and soy to farming wind. For increasingly, when we talk about making an omega-3-friendly world, we really are not just talking about food production. We're talking about the food-energy complex that, were it properly balanced, would prove to be as energy efficient as it would be metabolically healthy.

Currently the food-energy structure we have in place centers on the production of corn for animal feed and corn for ethanol fuel. The only reason farmers have turned to ethanol production is that the United States has engineered an unbalanced system that overproduces corn. The food system as it is simply cannot absorb any more. We have all the high-fructose corn syrup, processed food, and animal feed that we need. Ethanol is simply a way of handling the excess commodity crops. It is highly subsidized and highly wasteful. Currently around 40 percent of the corn grown in the United States is used to make ethanol. The ethics of using arable land to grow something for consumption by automobiles rather than by people have been hotly debated for more than a decade now. But no matter how you look at the ethics of the issue, for the average middle-American farmer the economics speak for themselves. The midwestern farmer is now intrinsically dependent on the energy economy to stay in the black.

But what if that energy slice of the farmer's pie was to come from something other than ethanol? What would happen if instead of harvesting corn, farmers let their land go back into carbon-storing grassland and learned to harvest the wind instead? Many positive things, it turns out.

Cliff Etheridge is a thoughtful septuagenarian former cotton farmer who is the organizing force behind the Roscoe Wind Farm, the largest wind-generating field in Texas. He is perhaps the biggest advocate there for a reimagining of the Great Plains. When I met him a little while back he gazed out over hundreds upon hundreds of windmills and proudly exclaimed, "This is the Texas way of dealing with this renewable situation."

Today landowners in the flatland around Abilene compete for lucrative wind royalties from European and even Chinese investors. When I first met Etheridge in the alternative-energy-friendly time of the early aughts, wind-rights telemarketing speculators were roaming the Greater Abilene White Pages, much in the same way that the "land men" of the 1940s oil boom wandered the Texas plains with blank oil leases. Etheridge took a more fair-minded, collaborative approach, building on existing ties with neighboring farmers, meting out carefully structured deals with Airtricity (the wind farm's Irish proprietor), and assembling a collective lease for one hundred thousand acres of land to host hundreds of towers. And his efforts are much appreciated in this impoverished swath of depopulating farming villages. If the surveyor's laser falls favorably upon your land in the emerging wind belt you may be compensated somewhere on the order of $13,000 per year per turbine. It is no surprise that Etheridge practically goes teary eyed, holding his buff white cowboy hat on his head while he tilts his head at the softly whirring turbines above. "I think they're just magnificent."

A switch away from a corn/soy/ethanol system to a Kernza/ pasture/wind system might well put farmers in a better place economically. But it would also diminish the overall amount of animal protein available to humans. And while it is true that around half of the protein increase anticipated by 2050 is merely an affluence effect of more people wanting to unnecessarily eat more animals rather than an actual need, the other half of that increase is the sheer population growth of individuals simply trying to get their 90 grams a day. Like it or not, pasture-raised animal systems, which would produce only 25 percent as many food calories as feedlot animals, won't get us to the protein levels we need.

Where would the additional food come from?

Right now, the balance of food production is heavily weighted toward the land. But there is an option to rebalance in the direction of the sea. As Steve Gaines pointed out, nearly every food we get from the sea is more resource efficient than what we grow on land. Catching wild fish, depending on the kind of fishing employed, can have a significantly lower carbon footprint than livestock production. But there is, of course, only so much wild fish available. We have to rethink, then, how we get food from the ocean.

Aquaculture—the farming of the sea—could make up the

protein difference. The problem is that until now, aquaculture has mirrored land food farming in the way it overuses resources. Modern-day fish farmers like to refer to the last century's surge in aquaculture production as a "blue revolution"—a marine reimagining of food production reminiscent of the food innovations that took place during the terrestrial green revolution. Until very recently, the blue revolution has based itself on the reduction of billions of smaller fish every year combined with industrially produced commodity crops to provide the bulk of farmed fishes' calories. Add to that the energy required to harvest, process, and ship wild forage fish, feed turns out to be the largest single environmental impact of aquaculture at present.

But changing this model is plausible. In fact, aquaculture is moving so quickly that it is hard to keep up. Around the world, on land and on sea, humans are finally chipping away at the barriers to sustainably producing marine protein.

The first and most obvious change would be to transition reduction industries from direct harvest of wild animals to the reprocessing of by-products. Only about 60 percent of the average commercially caught fish is fillet. The rest—the guts, the heads, the bones—is typically discarded, sometimes at great expense to the fish processing companies. In 2011 the U.S. Environmental Protection Agency fined Trident Seafood, one of the largest seafood producers in the world, $2.5 million and required $30 million in plant upgrades for dumping untold tons of fish offal into the waters of coastal Alaska. But much of this waste is reclaimable and could be used for both the production of supplements and the creation of fishmeal and oil for aquaculture.

All this was pointed out to me recently in the Alaskan capital of Juneau by a fish oil manufacturer named Sandro Lane. A frenetically inventive man who learned to cold-press olive oil as a youth while growing up on his family's farm in Italy, Lane made his way to Alaska in the 1970s, where he opened one of the state's first large-scale salmon smokehouses. Slowly he earned a reputation as the producer of high-quality, cold-smoked Alaska lox. His reputation prompted a visit by a camera crew and none other than Martha Stewart in 2000. During a lull in the smokehouse filming, Lane showed Stewart around the rest of his facility. He walked her through the discards part of the operation, where thousands of pounds of salmon offal and trimmings were being prepared for disposal. Looking at the ruby-red gurry sloughing down the chutes, Stewart turned to Lane and asked, "Can't you do something with all of this? There has to be some value in this waste." It was a good question, one that Lane had been contemplating for a long time. And when he started running the numbers, he realized that there was likely more value in the waste stream than there was going into his smokehouse. Within three years, Lane created Alaska Protein Recovery, a biotech company that utilized Alaska salmon processing wastes. From these by-products, he created a brand of natural fish oil supplements, which he launched nationally in 2007. This triggered a competitive race among seafood processors in Alaska to more fully utilize their waste streams and reduce seafood discards. Increasingly, other reduction companies are starting to follow suit. The Norwegian company BioMar now uses trimmings from traditional fisheries to account for as much as 41 percent of the fish oil in its feed. But discards still represent the minority of the marine ingredients in aquaculture feed. There are still a lot of guts out there going into the garbage.

Beyond reprocessing fish discards, there are more high-tech solutions to fixing the aquaculture feed problem. One of the most knowledgeable people in the alternative feed world is Rick Barrows, a rail-thin man who has spent most of his career trying to develop an ecologically sound aquafeed, first for the U.S. Fish and Wildlife Service and later for the U.S. Department of Agriculture. He did this partly out of a passion for seafood, but also partly out of necessity. When I told him that during my research I'd gone on an all-fish diet for a year, he laughed a sad laugh and muttered, "That's nothing. I've been on an all-fish diet for about the last ten years."

Barrows had developed in midlife a rare syndrome that prevented his body from metabolizing land food meats as well as corn and wheat. A passionate elk hunter who resides in the big-game-hunting mecca of Bozeman, Montana, Barrows at the time of our interview was no longer eating land animal flesh of any kind. This was a mixed blessing. "Now when I go out in the woods the elk and deer just surround me. They can't smell any meat on me. I think that's why they say the Native Americans used to do a meat fast before they went out on a hunt." He now finds his blood pressure at 80 over 61. "It's so low it's actually a problem."

Barrows remains convinced that an omega-3-rich diet can come to us through aquaculture, which is why he has been formulating feeds that have no fish in them at all. "Fish need nutrients, not ingredients" is his mantra. That is, DHA and EPA omega-3s are essential for fish health but not necessarily EPA and DHA derived from other fish. After studying a variety of ingredients, he has arrived at a formulation that includes as its primary omega-3 component the very thing from which omega-3s first sprang two billion years ago: phytoplankton.

Barrows has formulated a phytoplankton-infused fish feed for rainbow trout and assisted in bringing it to market for a small company called McFarland Springs Trout in the High Sierras of Northern California. Recently I made my way through that parched country at the end of the two-year California drought, a haze of wildfire smoke burning on the border with nearby Nevada. Down a gravel road I found David McFarland noodling around his trout raceway, getting ready to close up shop for the evening. When he asked what I'd like to eat for dinner, I suggested one of his trout. He put his dip net into the raceway and pulled out a rainbow of about three pounds, every bit as vibrantly colored as a wild trout.

It was very close in flesh quality and color to Atlantic salmon, and its EPA and DHA levels equaled or exceeded those of wild fish. The trout are a cross between steelhead trout, a sea-run fish close in genetics to a salmon, and a famous strain from Eagle Lake across the Nevada border. Those fish are known for the deep red color of their flesh. This characteristic is accentuated by the natural astaxanthin that occurs in the pigmentation of the algae Barrows has incorporated into the feed. Furthermore, Barrows and McFarland have found that eliminating fishmeal from aquaculture feed can have added health benefits. "Fishmeal is loaded with calcium and phosphorus," Barrows told me. "That will eventually prevent the fish from being able to take up trace amounts of copper they need. Their color will fade, their fins will erode. That's why farmed fish can look so nasty."

It seems, then, that we are just around the corner from a perfect omega-3 protein. So why aren't we all eating it?

"The problem is, it's expensive," Barrows explained. "If you look at pricing, it's the algae oil cost that's killing us." But need the price keep on killing a sustainable solution? As long as the aquaculture industry has reductionism at its disposal, innovations like Barrows's algae-based feed are victims of economy of scale. The forces of reductionism are powerful and date back to the nineteenth century. The algae industry is in its infancy, going back just a couple decades. For the algae business to grow, we have to decide as a society that it is worthy of subsidy and support. Only in this way can we get a sustainable feed system in place that will achieve its own economy of scale.

There are, however, major agricultural forces working toward their own solutions of growing omega-3s. Ultimately those forces could lead us into a brave new world of genetic engineering. Not far from Rick Barrows's Montana home, in a field north of Billings, a genetic experiment is taking place involving an organism every bit as invisible to the consumer as Peruvian anchoveta but every bit as important. Rapeseed, a plant that has traditionally been cultivated as an oilseed crop throughout Europe, has naturally high levels of short-chain alpha-linolenic acid. Like nearly all land plants, it lacks the ability to make long-chain EPA and DHA fatty acids. But rapeseed has a long history of modification. Scientists in Canada in the 1990s edited out a gene that gave the oil an unpleasant odor. Because the first plantings took place in Canada, a new name was conceived for the resulting product: canola, from the words "Canada" and "oil."

Now scientists are returning to canola plants and editing them once again, this time in a way that will radically change the farming of fish. As Willie Loh of the agricultural giant Cargill told me, a decades-long project of DNA modification is finally bearing fruit—or, well, actually, oil. Using gene inserts, in the last few years Cargill has managed to retool canola plants so that they can lengthen the fatty acid chain from simpler ALA forms to marine-style EPA and DHA. Where did these genes come from? Once again, phytoplankton have stepped in and given us the potential for a giant leap forward. The very genes that first gave phytoplankton the ability to radiate to the poles all those hundreds of millions of years ago are now being used to help EPA and DHA radiate into terrestrial agriculture. With this modification we may at last solve the bottleneck that has kept fish farming from expanding. We can now grow a synthetic source of omega-3s to meet that critical part of an aquacultured fish's diet without killing any wild fish.

But what about the rest of the diet consumed by farmed fish—the roughly 65 percent of feed that now derives from soy and other terrestrial plants? I would discover a potential workaround making its way to market when I visited the North

American heartland of salmon farming: the bays and inlets of Nova Scotia. Just outside Halifax I came upon a nondescript industrial building bearing the name Oberland Agriscience. Inside I found a NASA microbiologist named Greg Wanger tending to a giant pile of maggots.

Well, not maggots really, but *Hermetia illucens*, also known as black soldier fly larvae. Black soldier flies represent perhaps the most exciting new innovation in the world of aquaculture. What makes them particularly exciting is the way they close an egregious loop in our current food system. In any given year, North Americans throw out around half of all the food they produce. True, more and more of it is being composted in cities that have composting requirements. But municipal compost facilities are notoriously inefficient, and most rescued food waste simply ends up getting spread over the tops of landfills. Black soldier flies are the missing link in recycling all that discard. In eight days a pile of newly hatched soldier fly eggs will achieve a three-thousand-fold increase in mass, devouring anything from bruised apples to pizza crusts in the process. In sixteen days, they are ready to harvest. Because Oberland has licensed a technology that stabilizes food waste, discards can be gathered and stored long enough for the hungry larvae to scarf it all down.

After harvest the larvae can be transformed into a meal that is quite palatable to salmon and other farmed fish. They produce a high-grade protein that can be processed much in the way wild anchoveta are now used. "In trials we're seeing soldier flies being 98 percent as efficient as fishmeal," Wanger told me, adding with typical Canadian modesty, "That's pretty good!" The final element that makes soldier flies a slam dunk is that even though they are voracious as larvae, they are mouthless and ascetic as adults. They die at the first frost and are unlikely to survive if they escape and therefore pose little risk of becoming an invasive species. If the project expands to its full potential, yet another part of the current food system will become unnecessary and yet one more part of it will be transformed from an open-ended, wasteful affair into a closed loop. And lest the reader think this is a small, boutique solution, one need only look at the potential to see how truly revolutionary it could be. When I asked Wanger to do a quick calculation of the amount of soldier fly larvae that could be produced if we used all of North America's annual food waste of sixty million tons, he put the potential at twelve to sixteen million metric tons, more than three times the Peruvian anchoveta harvest. And if the excess cow manure that so toxically accumulates in lagoon ponds around the continent were ever to be incorporated into the black soldier fly feed base, Wanger estimates that we could grow *eighty million metric tons* of larvae—the weight of the entire catch of fish around the world. Reading that number back to himself, Wanger exclaimed, "Yowzers!"

There are even more fascinating and science-fiction-esque feed solutions around the corner. Researchers at the Norwegian University of Life Sciences have developed both yeast and bacteria that produce protein and fat profiles quite similar to fishmeal. Yeast can be grown on a substrate of lumber by-products. Bacteria can be produced on a plume of natural gas. Both of these microorganisms require only a fraction of the fossil fuels, freshwater, and land area as soy to come to market.

Proponents argue that these new forms of feed can be used to feed land animals as well as fish. But a fish ultimately has a much smaller carbon footprint than a land animal. That's because fish, unlike land food animals, are poikilotherms—cold-blooded. All the energy mammals and birds put into heating their bodies, fish put into building flesh. Fish also differ from land animals in that they do not need to expend energy to resist the pull of gravity—they float. All the energy land animals put into standing, fish can put into growing flesh. If tweaked in the right direction, fish really and truly could be the protein of the future.

And, actually, in the sea, we can do even better than fish. Because there is a whole class of plants and animals that comes from the sea that doesn't require any inputs at all. This was brought to my attention by Bren Smith in my home state of Connecticut.

A stocky, determined man born in Canada of American Vietnam War refuseniks, Smith was raised on the shores of Newfoundland (pronounced Canadian-correct with the emphasis on the "land"). His native waters were so cold he never bothered to learn how to swim. But he perversely continued to love the sea above all other passions. He eventually ended up in Alaska in the 1980s during the heyday of the American fishing boom. "For ten years I fished for McDonald's in Alaska," he told me. "I caught and killed *everything*. I was just a cog in a machine."

Disgusted by what he considered to be egregious destruction of the marine environment, he eventually made his way to coastal Connecticut, where he acquired several acres of bay bottom and started farming oysters. He loved the fact that oysters didn't require any feed (they subsist on filtering algae) and that a bottom full of shellfish tended to be restorative to marine ecosystems, cleaning and clearing the water while providing habitat for fish. The only problem was the hurricanes and major storms that have become increasingly commonplace in the northeast.

"Hurricanes Irene and Sandy both wiped me out," Smith explained. The two successive storms in 2011 and 2012 buried his oysters in their cages under tons of silt. The oysters suffocated and died, quite a loss for a crop that takes three years to grow. That's what led him to something he calls the arugula of the sea, better known to the rest of us as kelp. Kelp turns out to be even more restorative than oysters. One of the major problems coastal communities in heavily populated areas like Long Island Sound face nowadays is nutrification in the form of organic nitrogen. Just like the Gulf of Mexico, the sound is afflicted with seasonal dead zones that choke off life. Smith's kelp crop directly changes this dynamic. Kelp absorb nitrogen and incorporate it into their leaf structures. Once the kelp is harvested the nitrogen leaves the water column with it.

Many species of kelp can have significant levels of omega-3s, and some even produce protein. But apart from providing food for humans, kelp can also be fed to terrestrial animals. Cattle and other ruminants process kelp nearly as efficiently as they do grass. More significant for climate change, a recent study has found that cattle fed on kelp have markedly lower methane emissions. Though it might sound counterintuitive, someday kelp-fed beef could in part replace corn-fed beef.

But there is an even greater step we can take away from land. A step that, if we take it, might just address the worst problems of our food and energy systems.

An investigation of humanity's food future ultimately causes you to reflect on the past, and how through a series of accidents we distanced ourselves from our evolutionary roots in the sea. In the beginning we ate wild game, leafy greens, and seafood—a diet that put us in a one-to-one balance of omega-3s and omega-6s. In the next phase we tamed the wild grasses and bred them to produce grain and moved ourselves subtly in the direction of omega-6. Still a tolerable balance, but trending in an unfavorable direction. In the next and most recent phase we industrialized both grain and meat production and tilted ourselves to a way of eating and farming that is making us and our planet sick. But today we stand on the verge of another revolution—a revolution that will take us out to sea and, in a way, back to the very beginning.

Reflections like these came to me as I stood on a raft in the Bronx River estuary looking south toward the New York City skyline. On the raft with me was Gary Wikfors of NOAA's Milford, Connecticut, lab, the man who had first explained to me the origins of phytoplankton and omega-3s. The floating platform we were standing on was an experiment that Wikfors and others had launched the previous spring. Hanging beneath it were long, socklike nets that had been seeded with *Geukensia demissa*, commonly known as ribbed mussels. The point of the two-year experiment was to see whether mussels would survive or even thrive in the effluent that flows from New York into the ocean at large. If the mussels did in fact prosper in this environment, it could have implications for how we might help clean up coastal waters while creating omega-3-rich food.

The idea of using bivalves like mussels, oysters, and clams to purify waterways has been gestating for decades. In macro-ecological terms, mussels are the lower intestines of coastal river systems. Using a complex set of biological filters, they remove particulate matter from the water column, with a special talent for disposing of phytoplankton. In so doing, mussels can reduce some of the nutrient load coming into waterways from agriculture, wastewater treatment, and other anthropogenic sources.

Carter Newell, the founder of Pemaquid Mussel Farms in Damariscotta, Maine, who had joined us on the Bronx River raft, explained that mussels hung from rafts do something that other bivalves don't: they work in three dimensions. Mussel rafts, with their long ropes of ever-growing bivalves, can be established in 3-D, working throughout the water column at incredible densities and filtering large amounts of water.

"My mussel rafts are forty feet by forty feet," Newell told me. "That means they can filter something like five million liters of water per hour." The rafts also provide habitat. "I have counted thirty-seven different species of invertebrates living among the mussels on their culture ropes," said Newell. The next major advantage mussels have is the ease with which they can be grown. This is due in large part to the tremendous amount of wild mussel seed, called spat, that still swims in American waters.

Once they set and grow, mussels are also extremely hardy in surviving the kinds of extreme weather events we're likely to see in an era of climate change. Eva Galimany, a marine biologist with the Institute of Sciences of the Sea in Barcelona and a member of the team working on the NOAA project in New York City, said the sheer abundance of mussel species means that mussels are highly adaptable to a range of conditions. "From my experiments, they are great survivors, barely get sick, and can cope with many types of weather issues and toxins," she told me.

The problem, of course, is that not everyone will really want to eat mussels. At present bivalves are far down the list of Americans' most consumed seafoods. But that is where the other side of this organism comes in: mussels can make great food for the fish people do like to eat. Something that circles back to Scandinavia, the birthplace of reductionism and the very first omega-3 health studies.

For twenty years, the Swedish marine biologist Odd Lindahl had been looking at coastal pollution and getting sadder and sadder every time he thought of the monumental problems humans were creating. "I was fed up with creating negative headlines with new toxic blooms or new records in oxygen deficiency," he told me recently. "I wanted to do something positive, so I came in contact with a Swedish pioneer in mussel farming who had great visions of improving water quality by using mussel farming as a tool." This mussel farmer, a man named Juel Haamer, showed Lindahl how incredibly versatile these organisms could be. Together with Haamer, Lindahl applied mussel aquaculture to wastewater treatment plants, to coastal restoration, and to integrated polyculture systems. But by far the most valuable aspects of mussel culture are the protein and fats they can provide other animals. It is a high-quality protein that in animal feed "has the same result as fishmeal, and occasionally better," Lindahl told me. "And now we're finding we can put mussel protein in many things. In protein bars. In sausage. Even in ice cream. It's very versatile."

The only problem is, where do you put all those mussels? If shore owners don't want aquaculture in their backyards, where will the mollusks cause the least societal and environmental harm? This is where the last piece in the puzzle of an omega-3-leaning world gets interesting—and controversial. For it brings with it both the benefit of leading us to a major renewable energy source and the detriment of opening a new part of the ocean to exploitation.

Federally controlled offshore waters, usually beyond three nautical miles, have worlds of energy potential. Offshore wind is both stronger and more consistent than land-based wind and has the added benefit of blowing equally hard during day and night, including the afternoon, when energy demand is highest. True, offshore wind farms have been expensive to build. But just as with algae production, economies of scale play a role here. Larger offshore wind farms (that is, 500 megawatts per site or more) and farms built as part of a series are with each successive year being constructed for less cost. This in turn will allow developers to more quickly repay their investors. The United States can also now benefit from twenty years of expensive learning in Europe—something that has brought prices down to competitive levels. If offshore wind can be developed logically and with proper care to siting, the energy benefit to the country could be enormous. Willett Kempton, a professor at the University of Delaware's School of Marine Science and Policy within the College of Earth, Ocean, and Environment, noted to me that after he added up the wind potential of the American Atlantic, he was, well, blown away. "When we analyzed the U.S. eastern continental shelf, the permitting restrictions, and the wind speeds, we were astonished by the offshore wind resource size. It's enough to run the entire East Coast—electricity, vehicle fuels, and building heat. By comparison in usable power, the East Coast offshore wind resource is sixteen times greater than all East Coast offshore petroleum, deep- and shallow-water petroleum combined. We didn't expect that."

From a food systems perspective, a switch to wind power also circles back to a healthier diet. At present, about 30 percent of our energy comes from burning coal, which puts 24 percent of the world's anthropogenic mercury into the atmosphere. As seafood eaters well know, high levels of mercury in the blood have many health effects. These effects can range from change in behavior, compromised immune responses, autoimmune disorders, changes to the expression of reproductive hormones, and a limiting of a person's ability to respond to stress.

If we could replace coal-fired plants with wind generation, we would likely see a marked drop in methylmercury contamination. In U.S. waters, the shift from coal toward natural gas has already shown profound effects. When scientists measured mercury concentration in over twelve hundred bluefin tuna from the northeast Atlantic for an eight-year period from the 1990s to the early 2000s, they observed a 19 percent decline in methylmercury contamination. The authors of the study noted that "this decrease parallels comparably reduced anthropogenic mercury emission rates in North America and North Atlantic atmospheric mercury."

It's interesting to note that whenever I've brought up the subject of mercury contamination in seafood in the press, my inbox is quickly filled with messages from people in and around the tuna industry trying to assure me that the risk of methylmercury has been exaggerated. The element selenium, they insist, is present in most ocean fish, and since selenium bonds to methylmercury before it can bond to organic chemicals in the body, eating ocean seafood is safe for most consumers. What I never hear from the tuna industry is a complaint against coal. Where, one wonders, is the class action lawsuit of the fishing industry against the coal industry? Indeed, when I ask consumers why they don't eat seafood, high atop their reasons is that they are afraid of mercury contamination. Doing away with coal would go a long way toward solving that issue.

Coal and mercury aside, there is a still more interesting benefit of offshore wind power to a seafood diet. An offshore wind farm would provide anchoring structures for offshore aquaculture, something proposed most recently by the German researcher Bela Buck. Because wave energy is particularly intense beyond twenty nautical miles from shore, some kind of fixed anchoring structure would be critical in developing offshore aquaculture. The superstructure of a wind farm could do the job. Indeed, the joint investment food companies and energy companies could bring to a wind/fish collaboration could make the growth of this technology sector all the more plausible.

Currently most aquaculture operations are sited within a mile of shore where local opposition from coastal landowners is common. Anti-aquaculture activists maintain that excrement and uneaten feed pellets can accumulate under aquaculture pens and that this effluent can harm life on the seafloor below. Shore owners also don't like the idea of fish pens in their fields of vision.

But offshore, the picture is different. There is much more potential for dilution and distribution of waste from farms. Aquaculture and harmful algal bloom scientist Dr. Jack Rensel, who has worked with academics, government, and industry since 1974 and who co-heads a company that produces software to model the effects of fish farms, believes that "if there were large fish farms properly located and spaced in the open ocean, there is a huge capacity to assimilate the waste dissolved nitrogen into the food web without adverse perturbations."

Imagine, then: kelp farms inshore, processing nitrogen wastes and clearing waters of nitrogen loads so that coastal ecosystems start to recover from hypoxia. Imagine too, mussel and fish farms offshore where their ecological impacts would be minimized. Fish and shellfish that could offset the demand for industrial feedlot land food meat and all the environmental degradations those petroleum-intensive systems cause.

There are, of course, real dangers to moving forward with this next food revolution. As Gary Wikfors noted, "Any action we take as a species is going to take away from something else somewhere else." Many ocean conservationists flatly reject aquaculture. And they are right to be cautious about a major development of a bioregion that we don't yet fully understand. Aquaculture operations *do* risk overloading areas with nutrients, especially if farms are sited in areas of poor water flow. Antibiotics, carcinogenic antifoulants, and nitrate-heavy feed all risk throwing off the chemistry of surrounding waters. Even mussels, which don't require feed, excrete and can overfertilize an area if too densely concentrated. And any open-ocean aquaculture operation, be it fish or bivalve based, poses problems to wild fauna. Whales can become entangled in mussel ropes. Farmed fish can escape their pens and become a form of genetic pollution to other species around them.

But what is the alternative? The continuance of the giant experiment we've conducted on land? The terrestrial food systems of today eliminate biodiversity even as they load the atmosphere with carbon dioxide and methane; they are a major contribution to ocean acidification and dead zones; they use freshwater at a scale that cannot be sustained and that would be entirely unnecessary in an ocean-based model. In short, the industrial land food agriculture we rely on today is based upon a series of accidents—chance discoveries that were employed pell-mell with little thought to the collateral damage they would cause the environment. What would happen if we built a new system in the sea where we actually planned things?

Looking at all that potential, Wikfors shook his head. Back in his lab, we walked past darkened laboratories, shut tight from sequesters and budget squabbles while producers of corn and soy, beef and pork, continue to receive their annual

$15-billion-a-year subsidy. I asked Wikfors if all the fear about an ocean-based food system was warranted. Could we overload the system just as we did with land food?

"Honestly," he said, an optimistic grin on his face despite all sentiments to the contrary brewing in the world, "we have so little capacity right now. We don't even know what the limits are."

CONCLUSION

I write these closing words during the warmest and longest Indian summer I can remember. The average American temperature for September 2017 was 1.4 degrees above the twentieth-century average and among the warmest three in the historical record. The extreme heat in the ocean sent five hurricanes up from the Caribbean, four of which were classified as major. Coastal Texas, which has been robbed over the last two hundred years of its buffering wetlands by agriculture and real estate development, found itself under ten feet of water during the highest crest of Hurricane Harvey's storm surge. Meanwhile, NOAA, the agency that collected this data and that oversees all of the United States' fisheries and aquaculture programs, was facing a potential budget cut of 16 percent.

But amid this cacophony of catastrophe, there was one whisper of good environmental news that went largely unreported. Simply put, the late summer and early fall of 2017 saw one of the greatest resurgences of marine wildlife the American Atlantic coast has experienced since colonial times. This rebirth was spurred by the very fish I chased at the beginning of my omega journey aboard that Jet Ski in the Chesapeake Bay—the ignominious little oily fish called menhaden.

This renaissance was a long time coming. Over the course of the last century the principal catcher of menhaden in America, a Virginia-based company called Omega Protein, had morphed from a fertilizer company to a margarine and industrial oils maker to a terrestrial animal feed company to, most recently, a supplier of fish oil for omega-3 supplements and fishmeal for aquaculture. Annually it removes around three hundred million fish from the coastal Atlantic.

But beginning in the early 2000s a gradually emerging coalition of conservationists and fishermen began organizing around what the writer H. Bruce Franklin had deemed in a book of the same title "the most important fish in the sea." In 2010, after a long fight, the Atlantic States Fisheries Management Council concluded that menhaden were overfished and that fishing had to be cut by 20 percent.

By the fall of 2017, that 20 percent appeared to have flourished and propagated. In the wake of all that forage a host of predators stormed in. The Long Island–based writer and conservationist Carl Safina reported a changed sea. "This wasn't the ocean I've known all my life," he wrote. "This is a new and improved, revitalized coast, returning to abundance, where everything has plenty to eat and big things linger all summer getting fat and staying relaxed." Whales and dolphins had invaded a stretch of Block Island Sound that one local whale-watching company had previously dubbed "the dead sea." Now it was alive with menhaden and everything that ate it. Schools of thresher sharks, fifteen-foot whiptail creatures typically relegated to the distant offshore, blitzed the beaches of the East End, and osprey appeared to have increased their broods to three chicks per nest. Whales, chasing menhaden, breached in sight of the New York City skyline. Academics who had historically supported the reduction industry's positions argued that the resurgence of menhaden was not particularly related to a lowering of fishing pressure, and that environmental conditions could just as easily have led to the surge. But the conservation faction disagreed. "A blind man can see the impact," a local charter boat captain wrote to me from the Jersey shore.

Since the cutback, Omega Protein has fought hard to have its missing fish returned. In May 2015, I sat in on the Atlantic States Fisheries Management Council's meeting in suburban Virginia to watch the contest. In the center of the room a bloc of yellow-shirted Omega Protein workers testified as to why they should be allowed to up their catch. They cited jobs and economic health of the region. But when the discussion turned to whether more fishing would be *scientifically* advisable, the issue became thorny and entangled with the same bogeys that had dogged me all along in my omega journey: risk and uncertainty. Unlike a medical trial in which human subjects can be placebo-controlled and directly observed for effect, the natural world can only be modeled and risks only abstractly assessed. When Jason McNamee, the chairman of the technical committee that evaluated the menhaden question, presented a number of population scenarios with different rates of exploitation, he admitted that the possible outcomes swung wildly according to the rules of probability. "The projections are highly uncertain," he said. In response, a committee member named Louis Daniel posed an awkward question.

"Can you give some direction of the uncertainty, or is it just all over the place?"

"It goes in both directions," McNamee replied. "There is no easy answer to figure out which way the risk is."

This discussion of risk jostled loose another data point now permanently lodged in my head. Wasn't the prognostication for the reduction of risk of cardiac death through omega-3 supplementation sometimes estimated to be as low as 1 percent? Which risk did we want to take as a society? A slightly elevated risk of more people dropping dead of a heart attack? Or a much more unpredictable risk of hobbling an entire ecosystem, just because a single company wanted its additional thousands of tons of menhaden? And actually, in light of everything I'd learned about the myriad nonfish alternatives to menhaden and all the other little oily fish in the sea, it seemed it was a risk we didn't even have to take at this point.

These arguments have yet to sway the opinion of decision makers. In November 2017, just as I was putting the finishing touches on this book, the Atlantic States Fisheries Management Council met again to debate the issue. In spite of more than 150,000 public comments largely in favor of an approach that would more cautiously take into account the forage needs of other marine predators, the council ruled to delay action on legislating around the ecosystem role menhaden play. Ben Landry, Omega Protein's director of public affairs, didn't see anything wrong in that decision. "It's not a situation where we're *never* going to get ecosystem-based reference points," he told me. "It's just a couple years away. . . . We're not opposed to ecosystem reference points. We just want them to be menhaden specific." Omega wanted the menhaden judged on its own merits. Not lumped in together with the larger world of reductionism.

How this fight will go in the future depends, I think, on how much we imagine ourselves as parts of larger systems rather than isolated little existences and whether we decide to confront the very issues at the heart of reductionism. There is no better way to sequester carbon than to encourage a rich relationship among a multitude of carbon-based life forms. From hundred-foot whales to the half-inch krill they gulp down, from prairie grasses with root structures three yards deep to the wandering ruminants that browse upon them, these rich, diverse relationships balance the planet. They tie carbon down and put it to good use, rather than letting it make mischief in the atmosphere. Menhaden and all the living things in the world that are "reduced" today are part of that complexity. That we have not yet assessed those little oily fish at their proper value speaks, I think, of an immaturity on our part, rather than an insignificance on the part of the poor menhaden. At one point in history, we boiled down whales for margarine. Is boiling down menhaden for supplements any better? In a world we have pushed so far to an ecological brink is there *any* slack left for lives to be used in such a way? With technology offering us so many ways to close the loop of waste and to lead food production to so many new and more efficient directions, should we really continue to rely on practices that hail from the days of Melville?

As I contemplate all this, I realize that there is something about the holistic take on life that relates back to my own life and where I stand in the timeline of my particular journey. Once again I recall that odd map of the time zones of Antarctica—those arbitrary-colored pie segments different nations had assigned to prove their sovereignty in that last undiscovered country. Such divisions were laughable. In the unity and clarity of a single six-month-long Antarctic summer day, one sees the error in this kind of isolationist thinking. A way of thinking that we have erroneously applied not only to ecosystems but also to the structures of our very lives.

The subdividing of one's life into phases is exactly what those who take advantage of our insecurities are banking on. Whether it is a supplement company selling a remedy for compromised arteries or a car company trying to get you to upgrade from a compact to an SUV, all of them are trying to accomplish the same thing. They are trying to divide life into marketable sections, each with an array of products that fit a particular phase. The same was true of nutrients. The forty-year-old trying to build muscle mass at the gym is sold whey protein. The fifty-year-old is hawked omega-3s for his heart and failing mind, the sixty-year-old calcium for her bones. All of these nutrients in their own way are, of course, essential. But their value is only meaningful in the context of a larger system.

When I reflect on the funk that had driven me to the omega-3s in the first place, I realize that much of it is the result of my own misguided thinking. I had fretted over the looming threat of middle age and grown fearful that I had backed myself into a creative and professional corner. I had felt banished to the sea and seafood—a niche that occupied only a fragment of the average American's consciousness. I had wanted to move beyond the ocean and to explore and report on a much wider world.

But, funnily enough, my plunge into the most arcane subject the ocean had to offer—omega-3 fatty acids—had thrown a tether out to that wider world. That we were all born of the ocean and that we all carry the ocean in our cell membranes is something that I had passively known. But now I knew that this bond was much more intense and vital and played itself out in the millions of chemical bonds that coursed through my blood and my brain. Knowledge of this chemical connection brought into sharp relief the way we have misused land and sea alike and upset the equilibrium of the very climate upon which we depend. All this stirred a desire to make a struggle to regain this equilibrium central to the time I had remaining.

When I remembered all the people I'd met in my omega journey—the algae probers, the ice core drillers, the river monitors, the biotech synthesizers—I realized each was in his or her way engaged in that same struggle. Curiously, all of them were well into their forties, fifties, and sixties—in the omega end of their life's journey, if you will. All of these scientists and innovators were each very different, but they all shared one indubitable quality: they refused to believe in phases. For them, there was no "rind of life." From the early years of consciousness on through Indian summer, life was one whole fruit. By cultivating an appetite to eat through every layer of that fruit, skin and core and all, the people who most successfully maintained their vigor cultivated a celebration of life's complexity. The storms they encountered, the difficulties that threatened to level them—they approached them all with curiosity, a deep faith in the scientific method, and an unending belief in the necessity of forward momentum. Even in the face of cataclysm their central mission was to realize completely lived lives.

Only the truly unhealthy would look at their lives in terms of phases, each with their own diagnosable afflictions, curable by a single compound. The true antidote is careful, complex thought and full engagement—a constant, robust, sometimes futile-feeling striving toward balance.

EATING THE
FUTURE TODAY

No matter how far away an omega-3-centric world may seem, it is no further away from us than the bizarre and wasteful commodity crop/petroleum/reductionist system was from societies at the beginning of modern agriculture's last major shift. Imagine what a yeoman farmer from the early nineteenth century would have said if you described the plan for the next two hundred years: fossilized algae will be pumped from the ground and burned to create energy. Next a network of pipes will be laid under much of America's farmland to drain it of its excess moisture. Crop by crop, we'll pare down the bulk of what is grown until we focus on two species: corn and soybeans. Hardly anyone will eat these crops. We'll take all of the grazing animals off the land, put them in feedlots, feed them that corn and soy, and supplement their diet with a range of things including anchovies carted in from the Southern Hemisphere.

My guess is that no one would have found that to be a particularly plausible, let alone good, idea.

So the idea of a food system that could promote longer, healthier human lives, that recycles rather than generates pollution, and that has the potential to produce a whole coast's worth of energy—I don't think anyone would say that this was an unworthy goal.

But until the day when the food system starts to shift meaningfully in that direction, there are actions the average consumer can take to embrace an omega-3 world even if it's not here yet. Here, then, are some thoughts on eating that dream:

Eat a Mediterranean/Pesca-terranean Diet. What does eating a Mediterranean Diet mean? When I asked Walter Willett, one of the diet's most cited scholars, he put it very simply. "It's a whole package of healthy components: healthy forms of fat, whole grains compared to refined grains, a variety of fruits and vegetables, nuts, modest amounts of dairy, and low amounts of red meats. Put that all together and it basically describes the Mediterranean Diet." In the Pesca-terranean model, one would strive to make the animal protein portion of the diet as ocean-based as possible.

Try to get your omega-3s from food whenever possible. When I asked Gary Wikfors if any of his work at NOAA had influenced his personal eating habits, he replied very bluntly: "The first very practical aspect of my scientific knowledge that influences my own nutrition is to reject supplements. That comes from years of working with lipid chemists and algal samples and the precautions one has to take to avoid oxidation. No lipids are more prone to oxidation than omega-3s. Oxidation will result in the creation of cytoxic compounds." These compounds are, at best, not helpful to living cells. In an industry where much fish oil is still being harvested using vessels that lack necessary refrigeration, oxidation remains a problem.

Eventually it may be solved, but why even involve yourself in this industry in the first place? There is something to be said for the argument that a food should be eaten in context, and taking a lipid-based supplement outside the context of other lipids does seem to work against metabolic logic. In any case, just a little more than an ounce of canned anchovies is enough to meet the 500-milligram daily intake many physicians suggest for omega-3 consumption, though to this day there is no recommended daily allowance of omega-3s.

If you want to continue taking omega-3 supplements, take supplements that do not derive from fish caught specifically for reduction. There are several brands of marine oil that use by-products from fish for human consumption as their source. Among them, Pure Alaska Omega Salmon Oil and Wiley's Finest (derived from pollock discards) are worth considering as is good old-fashioned cod liver oil (Peter Möller's nineteenth-century cod liver oil company is still selling the stuff). Because the oil derives from fisheries that are already geared toward harvesting fish for human consumption, there's a better chance that the raw materials will have stayed under refrigeration throughout the supply chain, leading to a lesser chance of oxidation. There are also several brands of omega-3 supplements derived from algae that are currently on the market. Almega, Isaac Berzin's creation from Imperial, Texas, is intriguing because instead of using fermented sugarcane as a substrate to grow algae, the company relies entirely on photosynthesis-fueled algae. It's worth remembering that any omega-3 supplement regardless of its source is prone to oxidation. Supplements should therefore be kept under refrigeration.

Check your omega-3 level. While there will continue to be debates around taking omega-3 supplements, there does seem to be a fairly strong association between maintaining a healthy level of omega-3s in blood lipids and decreased risk of cardiovascular disease. It is now possible to determine the omega-3 level in your own blood. Several companies are currently active in this area. One, in Sioux City, South Dakota, is called OmegaQuant. For a modest fee that does not require a visit to a physician, OmegaQuant will send you a finger prick test and provide you within a few weeks with the lipid profile of your blood, including a detailing of your omega-3/omega-6 ratio.

Eat forage fish rather than fish fed on forage fish. Anchovies, herring, mackerel, and whiting are all fish that end up in the reductionist chain. Eating them directly is fully possible. With anchovies, look for cans labeled "product of Peru"—these are fish that would have been headed for the feed mills had not a few industrious entrepreneurs snatched a trifling 1 percent of the catch away from the reducers and prepared them for human consumption.

When eating aquacultured fish, look for aquaculture companies that favor innovation in feed. Farmed fish can reach a point where they are a more ecologically efficient form of protein than land food meats. Toward that end, try to look for brands that are focusing on reducing their use of forage fish and are innovating with their feed supply. Blue Circle salmon is one in particular that is using both algae-based products and offcuts from other fisheries to provide a significant part of their farmed salmon diet.

Eat mussels or other farmed bivalves. Mussels have a carbon footprint thirty times smaller than beef. At present Americans barely eat them. Increasing consumption will encourage an increase in production.

When eating land food meat and dairy, eat sparingly, and eat from grass-fed animals. It is probably unrealistic to wean every reader from meat altogether. But a stride toward better management of the planet would be to limit the amount of meat we eat in general to a few portions per month—the amount, by the way, recommended by the Mediterranean Diet. One gets even closer to the Mediterranean ideal if one favors pasture meat over feedlot animals. Grass-fed animals produce less methane and have a significantly lower carbon footprint. Grass-fed meat and dairy are also higher in omega-3s than feedlot animals, though keep in mind, their omega-3 levels are a fraction of those found in oily fish.

Support alternative energy development of all kinds. Of all the alternative energy prospects for the future, wind has the greatest potential, with something like twice the generating capacity of the next greatest provider, solar. Wind at sea blows hardest and most consistently and has the potential to provide the greatest energy return on investment. While various credible arguments have been made against offshore wind development (bird strikes, fish and marine mammal migration disruption, harmful vibrations, diminishing of the so-called viewshed), we must look at those objections in relation to the greenhouse gas emissions and ancillary pollution issues that arise from petroleum and coal. Moreover, because offshore wind establishes platforms for aquaculture development, it can potentially be the basis for an entirely new seafood-based economy.

Join an effort to take down a dam. Old dams currently block the migration of oily forage fish, particularly on the Atlantic coast. These largely useless dams from another industrial age artificially repress abundance and resilience and are also serious flood risks. American Rivers (www.americanrivers .org) is probably the most active national organization on dam removal, but local chapters of the Nature Conservancy, particularly in the northeast, work toward the goal of dam removal.

Support your local NOAA office. Because of its association with climate research, the National Oceanic and Atmospheric Administration might be one of the most beleaguered government agencies we have right now. Even before the present climate-change denialist government took hold in Washington, NOAA was a frequent target of budget reductions, suffering major across-the-board cuts during the government sequester. NOAA's Sea Grant programs are particularly worthy of support—both financial and moral. Recent budget proposals suggested zeroing out Sea Grant programs that provide education and technical assistance for aquaculture and other ocean-based industries. In the last two years these programs generated $575 million in economic impact and created or sustained more than twenty thousand jobs.

OMEGA IN THE KITCHEN

A decade ago, when I proposed my first book on seafood and the future of the oceans, I had a telephone conversation with a prospective editor at an old New York publishing house. All went very well and I was inclined to accept her offer. But then, just as we were signing off, the editor remembered she'd forgotten something.

"Will there be recipes?"

At the time this struck me as remarkably crass. Hadn't we just been discussing how fish are wildlife and not merely food? But as I reach the end of my third ocean book it occurs to me that I might have been a little too quick to judge. If I can't come up with any sustainable recipes, then what's the point of even trying to write about seafood?

So I'll take the opportunity here to share a few cooking ideas, items I've made for my family with good results. They come from a variety of sources. Some are adapted from my favorite cookbooks. Others are more improvisational. All of them are tweaked so as to maximize the omega-3 content. In a couple there is a little bit of dairy and in one a handful of cornmeal, perhaps to remind the reader that, in the Mediterranean tradition, one needn't banish land food from the plate. I've also included an oddball recipe at the end that you should *never* cook but that seemed so indicative of earlier times and curious old attitudes about wildlife that it merited inclusion.

I am not a professional chef, so take everything with this poor chef's grain of salt. None of these recipes has been "tested" (though my grammar school age son has proved an efficient screener for clunkers). Also keep in mind that these are not so much recipes as they are methodologies for approaching foods not typically eaten by Americans. Try one in place of a land food meat meal you might normally prepare. Riff upon them. Rename them. Make them your own.

Two-Can Sauce over Zucchini Linguine

This is a regular in our house. It is distinctly not fishy tasting, making it something I can get past my fish-averse son. It is an adaptation of Marcella Hazan's tomato and anchovy sauce from her brilliant *Essentials of Classic Italian Cooking*. I have tweaked it because Hazan's recipe with a scant four anchovy fillets doesn't carry enough omega-3 punch for a whole family. More important, I hate open cans sitting around in my refrigerator. Even more so now that I know omega-3-rich food left exposed to air will oxidize.

Here I recommend Peruvian anchoveta because it is the most commonly reduced fish in the sea—ground down for fishmeal and oil and seldom eaten. It is quite comparable to other anchovies, especially when incorporated into a sauce. For pasta I give an option here for "zucchini linguine." A relatively recent invention called a spiralizer transforms zucchini into noodlelike ribbons. Don't kid yourself—it's not pasta. But swapping spiralized zucchini for wheat pasta will dramatically decrease your carbohydrate load, something nearly all Americans could think about doing.

* SERVES 4

One 2-ounce can filleted Peruvian anchoveta packed in olive oil, reserve the oil

1 clove garlic

One 28-ounce can crushed tomatoes

4 zucchini, no more than 2 inches in diameter

Olive oil

Open the anchovy can and drain the oil into a medium-size saucepan. Chop the anchovies and mince the garlic. Set the heat to low. Fry the garlic for about 1 minute (don't let it brown). Turn the heat off and add the anchovies. Work the anchovies into the oil with a wooden spoon until they dissolve. Turn the heat back to medium. Empty the entire contents of the tomato can into the saucepan. Use a little water to rinse the rest of the tomato off the sides of the can and then pour that into the sauce. Cook uncovered on low heat for 30 minutes. Spiralize the zucchini. Just before you're ready to eat, you can either sauté the zucchini in 2 tablespoons of olive oil or, if you're trying to keep calories to a minimum, you may poach the zucchini directly in the sauce. If you choose the latter method, check that you have the right proportion of zucchini to sauce and remember that zucchini will continue to cook in the sauce even after you turn off the heat. Shoot to undercook it a bit if you're not serving immediately so that it is not mushy when it comes to the table.

Cauliflower Rice Paella

This recipe was conceived, again, to deliver high omega-3s but also to cut back on the carb load. It is basically a classic Spanish paella, heavy on mussels and squid (two omega-3 lodestars). I use a few shrimp, but mostly for the flavoring the shells and heads impart. The major switch here is cauliflower instead of rice. Cauliflower when pulsed through a food processor or grated over the large holes in a box cheese grater takes on rice-like qualities. It can be steamed or sautéed and carries only a fraction of the calories of rice.

* MAKES 4 APPETIZERS OR 2 MAIN COURSES

1 head cauliflower

½ pound whole shrimp, heads and all

3 tablespoons olive oil

1 onion, diced

1 clove garlic

1 fresh tomato, cubed

Pinch saffron

½ pound squid, cut into ¼-inch rings

1 pound mussels, scrubbed clean

Salt to taste

Grate or food process the cauliflower. Shell and head the shrimp. Put the shrimp shells and heads to boil in 1 cup of water. Meanwhile, heat the olive oil in a large pot over medium heat. Add the onion and sauté until translucent. Add the garlic and cook until just slightly cooked. Add the tomato and saffron. Cook for 1 minute, then add the squid. Cook on very low heat for 30 minutes. Once the squid is tender, add the cauliflower and sauté for 1 minute. When the cauliflower is hot, add the mussels. Toss and then pour the shrimp stock through a strainer into the pot. Cover and cook until the mussels begin to open (just a couple minutes). Roughly cut the shrimp bodies and add them to the mix. When the shrimp are cooked through, all the mussels should have opened, and your paella will be ready to serve.

Five-Minute Salmon

In survey after survey, Americans give three reasons why they don't eat more fish:

1. I don't want to touch it.
2. I don't know how to cook it.
3. I don't want it smelling up my house.

Because Americans feel so uncomfortable cooking fish, they are loath to spend a lot of money for something they might ruin. Here, then, my fellow Americans, is a recipe you cannot mess up.

In choosing the fish, my preference here is frozen sockeye salmon. Why sockeye? It is a bit lower in fat and calories than farmed salmon, often higher in astaxanthin (an antioxidant), and cooks faster (five-minute salmon, remember). It also has scales finer than farmed Atlantic salmon and can be cooked skin on without scaling. Why frozen? The bulk of wild

Alaskan salmon are caught from late June through about mid-August. When supermarkets display glistening wild salmon fillets outside of those months, they are usually previously frozen. Their quality is probably worse than the frozen portions in the freezer section and, oddly, the defrosted fish is often priced higher. The frozen fish tucked away in vacuum-sealed packets in the freezer section, meanwhile, is typically frozen so quickly after capture and at such low temperatures that there is almost no loss in quality. Supermarkets often have frozen packets that price out under $10 a pound.

• SERVES 2

Two 4-ounce portions sockeye salmon, skin on
Salt and pepper

Defrost the salmon in their plastic packets. (Ideally, put them in the refrigerator the night before. If you forget, they'll defrost in about 10 minutes submerged in water at room temperature.) When you're ready to start cooking, put a broiling pan on the highest rack in your oven and set the broiler to high. Blot the salmon dry. Sprinkle the meat side of the fillet liberally with salt and pepper. Put the salmon on the broiling pan skin side up. Cook for 5 minutes or until the skin begins to blacken and bubble. Serve immediately atop your favorite dark leafy green.

Sardine Butter

My family eats a lot of fish for breakfast and sometimes tires of the usual smoked salmon on a bagel. This recipe is an intriguing alternative and is especially good when served with a sharp-tasting vegetable like green onions or shallots. It is also a ridiculously easy thing to make. I use butter from pastured animals because dairy products from cows fed on grass can be significantly higher in omega-3s than dairy from feedlot cows.

* MAKES 4 TO 8 SERVINGS
One 4-ounce can sardines
4 tablespoons pasture butter, softened at room temperature
1 teaspoon lemon juice
Salt and pepper to taste
Green onion or shallot for garnish (optional)

Empty the entire sardine can with oil into a food processor along with the butter and lemon juice. Blend until smooth. Taste to check for salt. Add more salt if necessary and pulse once more. Press into ramekins, cover with wax paper, and refrigerate for at least 1 hour. Serve with good bread and garnish with scallions or shallots.

Kelp Pad Thai

A certain section of the food politics crowd is very interested in kelp, but very few know exactly what to do with it. An exception is Adam Geringer-Dunn, the founder of the Greenpoint Fish and Lobster Company in Brooklyn. Here, land food wheat noodles are replaced with strips of kelp. The result is delicious and low calorie.

* SERVES 4

Kelp Noodle Sauce

2 tomatoes

2 red Fresno chili peppers

2 cloves garlic, peeled

½ cup toasted sesame oil

¼ cup tamari

¼ cup liquid tamarind
    (available at Indian grocers)

¼ cup fresh lime juice

Kelp Noodle Mix

1 pound kelp noodles
    (can be purchased at higher end supermarkets like Whole Foods as
    well as some Asian specialty stores)

2 scallion tops, julienned

½ cup snow peas, julienned

½ cup carrots, peeled and julienned

½ red bell pepper, seeded and julienned

Garnish

½ teaspoon whole unsalted peanuts

½ teaspoon toasted black and white sesame seeds

Pinch fresh cilantro

Pinch salt

2 lime wedges

Place all the ingredients of the kelp noodle sauce in a blender and blend until smooth. Keep refrigerated while you prepare the noodle mix. Make a few rough cuts through the kelp noodles with a knife or scissors, just to break them up a bit. Rinse with cold water, then drain thoroughly. Mix the noodles with the kelp noodle sauce along with the scallions, snow peas, and julienned carrots and bell pepper. Put in a serving bowl and sprinkle with the peanuts, sesame seeds, cilantro and salt. Provide your dinner guests with lime wedges for spritzing.

Salmon Meatballs

Unlike typical meatballs, which are fried first to bind the ingredients, these are baked. Flaxseed and a free-range egg do the binding job, and the result is a light, high-omega-3 dish that is much lower in calories than red meat or pork. If served over spiralized zucchini instead of pasta, the meal is entirely gluten free.

• SERVES 4

Sauce

One 28-ounce can crushed tomatoes

2 tablespoons olive oil

Salt to taste

Salmon balls

12 ounces boneless and skinless salmon

½ cup milled flaxseed

1 pasture-raised egg

2 tablespoons onion

2 tablespoons Parmesan cheese

2 tablespoons parsley

2 tablespoons olive oil

Salt to taste

Preheat the oven to 400°F. Combine the tomatoes and 2 table-spoons of the oil in a deep baking dish and put into the oven un-covered. While the sauce is warming and reducing, put the salmon in a food processor and pulse until coarsely ground. Com-bine the ground salmon and all of the remaining ingredients in a bowl large enough to allow mixing by hand. Mix until all the ingredients are uniformly blended. If the mixture feels too moist to form into a ball, add more flaxseed meal; if too dry, add a little more oil. Form balls that are 2 inches in diameter and put them into the baking dish with the sauce. Cover the baking dish and cook for 15 minutes. Remove from the oven and turn the balls once. Bake for another 5 to 10 minutes. Serve over pasta, rice, or spiralized zucchini.

Anchovy Potatoes

This is another very unfishy fish dish that you needn't warn fish haters about. It also, like all my recipes, makes use of the entirety of the package of ingredients required so you don't have to worry about half-used cans or orphaned potatoes in your fridge. If you have leftovers they make a great lunch garnish the next day.

* SERVES 10

⅓ cup olive oil

One 5-pound bag potatoes

One 2-ounce can Peruvian anchovies, ideally packed in olive oil

Preheat the oven to 400°F. Put the oil in a large deep nonstick baking pan and put the pan in the oven during preheating. While the oven is warming, slice the potatoes into ¼-inch-thick half-moons. You may leave the skins on if you like. I prefer to have the additional nutrients the skins provide. Blot dry if you have time. Chop the anchovies finely. Remove the baking pan from the oven and put it on your stovetop. Add the anchovies and mash them in the oil with a wooden spoon until they dissolve. Add the potatoes and toss with the oil/anchovy mixture. Bake for about 90 minutes, turning every 15 minutes to ensure that potatoes are evenly browned.

Mussel Po' Boy

Most Americans associate the po' boy with oysters, but this southern sandwich can be done with mussels at about a quarter of the price. Chatham, Massachusetts, produces a large blue mussel of superior quality. Taylor Shellfish farms in Washington State grows a "Med" mussel that is also large, luscious, and wonderful.

* MAKES 3 TO 6 SANDWICHES

2 pounds large mussels

Canola or olive oil for frying

1 free-range egg

¼ cup milk from pastured cows

Salt and pepper to taste

¼ teaspoon turmeric

Cornmeal

Whole-wheat baguettes

Olive-oil-based mayonnaise

Put about ¼ inch of water in a large pot on high heat. When the water is steaming, add the mussels. Cook until they just begin to open. Here you are trying not to cook the mussels through—you want them still tender so that the frying part doesn't overcook them. Set the mussels aside to cool. Heat the oil to 375°F for frying. When the mussels are cool enough to handle, pluck the meat from the shells and set in a colander to drain. Beat the egg, milk, salt, pepper, and turmeric together. Dip the mussels in the egg mixture, then dredge them in cornmeal. Fry until they are golden and drain on paper towel. Serve on warm baguettes with olive-oil-based mayonnaise.

Glasmastarsill, or Glassblower's Herring

Around 80 percent of the Maine herring catch is used for lobster bait. Maine "sardines" (actually herring) used to be a large part of the state's economy, but after Clean Water Act regulations forced coastal canneries to close, herring were redirected into the bait market. So much herring bait is in the water in lobster traps that some now refer to the Gulf of Maine as one giant lobster farm. Bait slips through the cracks of lobster traps and feeds an ever-growing crop of baby lobsters. Lobsters in turn prey on juvenile codfish and haddock, repressing those overfished species. This practice has in effect turned the Gulf of Maine ecosystem upside down, where crustaceans instead of higher predators sit atop the web of life. A corrective to this would be to eat Maine herring instead of feeding them to Maine lobsters. And there's good reason to. Herring are extremely nutritious, high in omega-3s, and low in energy cost to catch. For someone of Jewish heritage there's even some poetic justice to it all. Herring is the ultimate kosher fish. Lobster is *trayf.*

So here's a way to make some of that herring go into human rather than lobster mouths. This recipe hails from Sweden and is typically served on Christmas. The lemon wedges and red onion give it a beautiful glow, and the low sugar means that the dish is more savory than the sickly sweet Jewish versions.

*YIELDS ABOUT 2 MASON JARS

5 cups water

¼ cup kosher salt

1 pound herring fillets

¼ cup sugar

2 cups white wine vinegar

1 teaspoon mustard seed

2 teaspoons whole allspice

2 teaspoons black peppercorns

3 bay leaves

3 whole cloves

1 lemon, thinly sliced

1 medium red onion, thinly sliced

Heat 4 cups of the water, hot enough to dissolve the salt. Let the brine cool to room temperature. When it does, submerge the herring in the brine and refrigerate overnight, or up to 24 hours. Meanwhile, bring the sugar, vinegar, the remaining cup of water, and all the spices to a boil. (Divide the spices between your containers if you are using more than one.) Simmer for 5 minutes, then turn off the heat and let this steep until cool. When the herring have brined, layer them in a glass jar with the sliced lemon and red onion. Pour the cooled pickling liquid into the jars and then seal them. Wait at least a day before eating. Store in the fridge for up to a month. Note: Herring fillets typically have bones in them but don't worry. The fine bones will soften in the vinegar mixture and will be unnoticeable in the final product.

Pink Salmon Melt

To this day I do not know why Americans will eat canned tuna by the pallet and yet eschew canned salmon with a vengeance. Although the sorts of tuna used for canning are not giant predators like Atlantic bluefin or bigeye, they are still alpha predators, consuming fish that have in turn consumed other fish or crustaceans further down the food chain. Skipjack, albacore, and the other canning tuna can thus bioaccumulate methylmercury when it passes from one food-chain level to the next. Meanwhile, sockeye and pink salmon, the salmon most commonly used for canning, feed mostly on small crustaceans and microscopic plankton. Their pinkish-orange flesh is in fact a direct result of the pigments from crustaceans. These salmon are as high if not higher in omega-3 fatty acids as tuna but bear none of the mercury risks. They also have significant amounts of astaxanthin. You can substitute canned salmon for any tuna recipe. Here I favor pink salmon because it is cheaper and comes in large enough cans to make salmon salad for a large lunch party.

* MAKES 2 TO 4 OPEN-FACE SANDWICHES

One 8-ounce can pink salmon

¼ cup yogurt

3 tablespoons onion, chopped fine

3 tablespoons celery, chopped fine

Juice ½ lemon

Rye bread

Cheddar cheese from pastured cows

Turn on the broiler. Combine the salmon, yogurt, onion, celery, and lemon juice. Spread over the bread, cover with the cheese, and toast under the broiler until the cheese has melted (3 to 5 minutes).

Roulades of Antarctic Penguin Breast

Never make this recipe, please. I include it here only as an artifact. It came to my attention at Port Lockroy, Antarctica, a research station once run by stalwart scientists known as FIDS (Falkland Island dependents). The *Fit for a FID Cookbook* was written by Gerald T. Cutland, who served as a general assistant/cook in the 1956–57 season on the Argentine islands just north of the White Continent. The book has a samizdat feel to it, and it often devilishly details how scientists made use of local fauna in the kitchen when they could not stomach another can of split peas. The cookbook is full of sage advice. When cooking a seal steak, for example, a chef should "make sure that all the blubber has been removed as blubber is one of the things that gives it that peculiar flavour which is not desirable." Cutland penned several penguin recipes, though he confessed that he was not a fan of the bird on the plate, noting, "I have an awful feeling inside of me that I am cooking little men." The book went on to be issued to every British base in Antarctica. Here is one of Cutland's more memorable penguin preparations.

Penguin breasts as required

Salt and pepper to taste

Rashers of bacon

Parsley or mixed herbs

Beef suet

1 cup reconstituted onion

2 tablespoons vinegar

1 tablespoon flour

Cut the meat into rectangles. Season with salt and pepper. Lay a rash of bacon on each and sprinkle with parsley. Roll up and tie with thread. Melt the suet in a pan and fry the rolls lightly until brown all over, and place in a baking dish. Fry the onion next and toss over the meat rolls in the baking dish. If desired, a few tomatoes may be added. Add water and the vinegar to the remaining fat in the pan. Bring to a boil and thicken with flour. Blend with a little water. Spoon over the meat rolls and cook in a moderate oven until the meat is tender, approximately 2 hours. When cooked, remove the thread and arrange the balls on a dish. Spoon gravy over and around the balls and serve with creamed potatoes and baked tomatoes. The gravy may be seasoned to taste.

Acknowledgments

ooks have a way of becoming chapters in the life of a
writer, and so a book's completion often marks a passage
to a new part of a larger narrative. Nevertheless, there
are recurring characters who play significant roles within and
without the march of texts, from the first early attempts at
composition on through an author's Indian summer and, one
hopes, beyond. For these informed and informing people I am
deeply grateful.

As always I must thank my good friend and continual con-
sigliere, Carl Safina, for the way he shares his love of the written word and the natural world. Both loves are infectious and
instructive.

Among my many sources a few need singling out for the ed-
ucational role they played in helping me trace the larger arc of a
bendy and difficult set of compounds: NOAA's Gary Wikfors
for his explanations on how omega-3s may have emerged during
the earth's early life; Patricia Majluf, formerly of the Peruvian
Ministry of Fisheries, now vice president of Oceana Peru, for her
guidance in understanding the ups and downs of the Peruvian
anchoveta fishery; the Global Organization for EPA and DHA
Omega-3s (GOED), with particular appreciation for GOED's

executive director, Ellen Schutt, for being my liaison with numerous physicians and manufacturers in the omega-3 universe; Dr. William Harris of OmegaQuant for walking me through blood lipids and how to go about measuring them; Dr. Jørn Dyerberg for sharing his experience with Greenland Inuits and the subsequent epidemiological history of omega-3s; Captain Joe Hibbeln, MD, of the National Institutes of Health for his insights into omega-3s and neurochemistry; Dr. Artemis Simopoulos for her explanations of the omega-3/omega-6 ratio; Professors Marion Nestle and Sarah Tracy for guiding me through the life of Ancel Keys and the research around the Mediterranean Diet; Professor Alex Purves at the University of California at Los Angeles for assistance in identifying key thinkers in the field of classical food studies; Paul Hartfield of the U.S. Fish and Wildlife Service in Jackson, Mississippi, for his instruction on the ways of the Mississippi in particular and of moving water in general; Beatrice Ughi and Danielle Aquino Roithmayr of Gustiamo for their ongoing tutorials on good food and better living; Professor Cassandra Brooks, John Weller, and Professor Lesley Thorne for their insights on the Antarctic Treaty and the fisheries history of the Southern Ocean; and Dr. Richard Shepard, my family physician, who gamely drew my blood and discussed fatty acids ad nauseam with me while I lay prostrate on his examination table.

The reader of endnotes will notice my reliance on a handful of key texts. Susan Allport's *The Queen of Fats* was central to my understanding of the chemical underpinnings and physiological roles of omega-3 polyunsaturated fatty acids. H. Bruce

Franklin's landmark work, *The Most Important Fish in the Sea*, drew my attention to the history of reductionism in North America, with a particular emphasis on Atlantic menhaden. It was Bruce who first made the connection between reductionism and supplementism and all the consequences that relationship entails. Callum Robert's *The Ocean of Life* traced a thread from early ocean evolution through Roman garum and on into the complex webs of marine ecosystems. Alanna Mitchell's *Seasick* gave a clear and deft review of the many diseases afflicting the body of the ocean. Michael Pollan's *The Omnivore's Dilemma* and *In Defense of Food* were essential in decoding the way Western societies industrialized agriculture and animal husbandry; D. Graham Burnett's *The Sounding of the Whale* coolly and correctly plumbed the horrible depths of the great Southern Ocean whale holocaust; Jill Santopietro's as-yet-unpublished (why?) disquisition on Mediterranean anchovies and the family of ancient fish sauces that seasoned classical tables brought the deep past to the present culinary moment. I must also single out the work of Mark Kurlansky, an author who continues to be an intellectual guide and source of inspiration in much of my writing. "It has always seemed to me that there were two ways of looking at things," Kurlansky wrote to me in the heat of battle with the present work. "You can either look at the broad subject and narrow it down or you can look at the narrow subject and explore its broad implications. . . . I tend to see great importance in small things." Amen to that.

More and more, the writing of books of a global nature requires the marshaling of forces beyond the world of books.

For material support during the research and writing of this project, a Pew Fellowship in Marine Conservation was indispensable, as was the Pew Fellows' intellectual community so wisely curated by that program's director, Polita Glynn. An ongoing Safina Center writer-in-residence stipend was also critical for support during the writing period. The Walton Family Foundation backed my early investigations into life on the Mississippi. And thanks are also due to Sven Lindblad and Lindblad Expeditions for granting me passage aboard their vessel *Explorer* to the Antarctic Peninsula.

A portion of the reporting for this book occurred concurrently with the filming of a PBS *Frontline* documentary called "The Fish on My Plate." Throughout much of the writing process I was lucky to have the ongoing editorial advice of *Frontline*'s brilliant, preternaturally empathic creator, David Fanning. Along with David, the film's director, Neil Docherty, and co-producer, Sarah Spinks, were sage advisers. In this vein I must also thank the Food and Environment Reporting Network (FERN) for its support of my coverage of the intersection of agriculture and marine/aquatic ecosystems for *The American Prospect* and *Eating Well* magazines. FERN's executive director, Sam Fromartz, was profoundly helpful in the editing of those land-based investigations.

On the larger editorial front I owe a bow of gratitude to my long-suffering editor, Emily Cunningham. Who would have thought that such small fish and tiny molecules would require so many drafts? Emily did the greatest service any editor can do for an author—saving him from his own literary pretensions. Carolyn Hall, my researcher, fact-checker, sounding board, and overall aide-de-camp, deserves special recognition for her combination of intellectual acuity and creative sense of flow. And thanks, of course, to David McCormick, my agent through the writing of what is now a marine trilogy. There would have been nary a fish book were it not for David's expansive vision and allegiance during this decade-long campaign. In that larger campaign I am also indebted to Ann Godoff and the Penguin Press for seeing me through my investigations from thousand-pound bluefin to microscopic dinoflagellates.

Thanks to David Gold, Tara Smith, Katie Baldwin, David Thorne, Clare Leschin, Rachel Othmer, Adam Bendixson, Nancy Harmon Jenkins, Zach Brown, Jane Black, Martina Pavlicova, Alex Star, Peter Hoffman, Ben Halpern, Phil Drill, Harvey Greenberg, Sharon Messitte, Nick Messitte, and all my other colleagues, friends, and family who reviewed the work-in-progress in tattered bits and broken pieces.

And last, thanks to the members of my closest cohort group: Esther, Tanya, and Luke—multivalent, statistically robust, ever changing, protective, you are the dynamic bonds that keep me feeling young even though some might suggest I have entered the omega end of my life.

Notes

EPIGRAPH

ix **"It goes into your body"**: From an omega-3 supplement user survey commissioned by BASF and conducted by Judy Taylor. Judy Taylor, "The Omega-3 Trust Paradox," filmed at the GOED Exchange 2016 Conference, Tenerife, Canary Islands. Uploaded March 4, 2016, video, 30:39, www.youtube.com/watch?v=WCqZjOVlgB8&list=PLHYxROoZNvQyKkhGq5d2_u_E890w8USXC&index=29.

INTRODUCTION

1 **million fish into medicine**: The vessels I was seeking were fishing for Atlantic menhaden on behalf of the Omega Protein Corporation, a reduction company based in Houston. In 2016, Omega Protein caught roughly 134,700 metric tons of menhaden. At approximately one pound per fish that would equal 301 million fish. Caught over the course of a season that translates into around 2 million fish a day. Ben Landry, Omega Protein's director of public affairs, confirmed in a December 15, 2017, conversation that vessel capacity is about a million fish. Catch statistics on menhaden can be found at "Atlantic Menhaden," Atlantic States Marine Fisheries Commission, www.asmfc.org/species/atlantic-menhaden.

3 **Salt Lake City called GOED**: Organized in 2006, GOED is a nonprofit trade association comprised of more than two hundred member and affiliate member organizations. Its mission is to "increase consumption of omega-3s to adequate levels around the world" through education and accountability for ethical and quality standards.

4 **"help prevent coronary heart disease"**: "Omega-3 Fatty Acids and Coronary Heart Disease," *Health Encyclopedia,* University of Rochester Medical Center, www.urmc.rochester.edu/encyclopedia/content.aspx?contenttypeid=1&contentid=3054.

4 **"increase brain volume"**: Julius Goepp, MD, "Omega-3 Fatty Acids Increase Brain Volume," *Life Extension,* August 2010, www.lifeextension.com/magazine/2010/8/omega-3-fatty-acids-increase-brain-volume/page-01.

4 **"boost sperm competitiveness"**: Annie Harrison-Dunn, "Plenty More Fish in the Sea: Omega-3 May Boost Sperm Competitiveness," Dairyreporter.com, September 28, 2014, www.dairyreporter.com/Article/2014/09/29/Omega-3-may-boost-sperm-competitiveness.

4 **"build muscle in older adults"**: "Omega-3s May Help Older Adults Build Muscle," Nutrition Express, www.nutritionexpress.com/showarticle.aspx?articleid=884.

4 **"prevent some forms of depression"**: "Omega-3 Fatty Acids May Prevent Some Forms of Depression," *ScienceDaily,* October 1, 2014, www.sciencedaily.com/releases/2014/10/141001090103.htm.

4 **"help lower risk of type 2 diabetes"**: Tracey Walker, "Omega-3s May Help Lower Risk of Type 2 Diabetes," *Formulary Watch,* Modern Medicine Network, January 27, 2014, http://formularyjournal.modernmedicine.com/formulary-journal/content/tags/diabetes/omega-3s-may-help-lower-risk-type-2-diabetes.

5 **of the human brain's weight**: Writing in the journal *Nutrients,* M. J. Weiser, C. M. Butt, and M. H. Mohajeri maintain that "over half of the brain's dry weight is comprised of lipids, and it is

especially enriched in long-chain omega-3 (n-3) polyunsaturated fatty acids (PUFAs), suggesting a key role for these molecules in the optimal development, maturation and aging of neural structures and networks. . . . DHA makes up over 90% of the n-3 PUFAs in the brain and 10%–20% of its total lipids. DHA is especially concentrated in the gray matter." If we do the math and assume that 50 percent of the brain's weight is lipid based and 10 to 20 percent of that 50 percent is DHA, that's a pretty hefty proportion for one molecular component. Quotes from M. J. Weiser, C. M. Butt, and M. H. Mohajeri, "Docosahexaenoic Acid and Cognition Throughout the Lifespan," *Nutrients* 8, no. 2 (February 2016): 99.

5 **taking the golden pill:** GOED's president, Adam Ismail, in a recent interview cited studies concluding that omega-3 supplementation was associated with a 9 to 30 percent reduction in risk of cardiovascular disease; Adam Ismail, "What *Frontline* Didn't Say About Omega-3s," New Hope Network, January 16, 2016, www.newhope.com/idea-xchange/defense-omega-3s. Most influential in showing cardiovascular effect was the GISSI-Prevenzione trial studying 11,324 participants with previous myocardial infarctions and comparing treatment with one fish oil capsule per day (850–882 mg EPA plus DHA as ethyl esters) with or without vitamin E, vitamin E alone, or nothing—all with the current standard of care—for 3.5 years. At the study's conclusion, the reductions in risk of total death and sudden death were significant. The authors concluded the lowered risk of all-cause mortality was driven primarily by the reduction in sudden cardiac death and hypothesized an antiarrhythmic effect of EPA and DHA. Neil J. Stone, "The Gruppo Italiano per lo Studio della Sopravvivenza nell'infarto miocardio (GISSI)-Prevenzione Trial on Fish Oil and Vitamin E Supplementation in Myocardial Infarction Survivors," *Current Cardiology Reports* 2, no. 5 (September 2000): 445–51.

5 **"was not associated with":** The *JAMA* study referenced is often referred to as the Rizos study. E. C. Rizos et al., "Association Between Omega-3 Fatty Acid Supplementation and Risk of Major Cardiovascular Disease Events: A Systematic Review and Meta-analysis," *Journal of the American Medical Association* 308, no. 10 (September 2012): 1024–33.

5 **Omega-3s already ranked:** One of the many rosy predictions for the omega-3 industry asserts that: "Global Omega-3 Market Growing at a CAGR of 7.57% Between 2016–2013," press release, MarketResearchReports.biz, September 28, 2017, OpenPR, www.openpr.com/news/745266/Global-Omega-3-Market-Growing-At-A-CAGR-of-7-57-Between-2016-2023.html. GOED suggests that overall sales of omega-3 products are around $30 billion annually.

6 **most studied organic molecules:** Omega-3s have some 574,000 references on Google Scholar, similar to vitamin B12 (558,000 citations), statins (406,000), and acetaminophen (326,000).

6 **fastest-growing food system:** Many sources cite aquaculture as the fastest-growing food system on the planet, though the UN Food and Agriculture Organization qualifies this statement with a "probably." Whether a "probably" is merited, it is clearly the fastest-growing form of animal husbandry. "Aquaculture," FAO, www.fao.org/aquaculture/en/.

6 **They create half:** John Roach, "Source of Half Earth's Oxygen Gets Little Credit," *National Geographic News,* June 7, 2004, news.nationalgeographic.com/news/2004/06/0607_040607 _phytoplankton.html. For the amount of carbon passing through phytoplankton, see Paul Falkowski, "Ocean Science: The Power of Plankton," *Nature,* www.nature.com/articles /483S17a?message-global=remove.

6 **It contains four times:** Elizabeth Pennisi, "Meet the Obscure Microbe That Influences Climate, Ocean Ecosystems, and Perhaps Even Evolution," *Science,* March 9, 2017, www .sciencemag.org/news/2017/03/meet-obscure-microbe-influences-climate-ocean-ecosystems -and-perhaps-even-evolution.

7 **reduce planktonic sources of omega-3s:** S. M. Hixson and M. T. Arts, "Climate Warming Is Predicted to Reduce Omega-3, Long-Chain, Polyunsaturated Fatty Acid Production in Phytoplankton," *Global Change Biology* 22, no. 8 (August 2016): 2744–55.

7 **equivalent of the human weight:** I arrived at this comparison in the following manner:
Current U.S. population: 326 million.
Current average weight of Americans: Men, 195 pounds; women, 162 pounds.
Assuming that roughly half the American population is men and the other half women, that gives a total human weight of the United States as 58.8 billion pounds. Forage fish extraction in 2006 took 23.8 million metric tons, which equals 52.5 billion pounds. Thus the U.S. human weight is roughly equal to the annual global extraction of forage fish for reduction.
    As a side note of interest, the weight of the average American woman is now equal to the weight of the average American man in the 1960s. Male American weight has grown similarly

heavy in the last half century, with men now weighing fifteen to twenty pounds more today than in the 1960s.

Sources: "U.S. and World Population Clock," United States Census Bureau, www.census. gov/popclock/; Christopher Ingraham, "The Average American Woman Now Weighs as Much as the Average 1960s Man," *The Washington Post*, June 12, 2015, www.washingtonpost.com/news /wonk/wp/2015/06/12/look-at-how-much-weight-weve-gained-since-the-1960s/?utm_term=.487349b1c19b; Albert G. J. Tacon and Marc Metian, "Fishing for Feed or Fishing for Food: Increasing Global Competition for Small Pelagic Forage Fish," *Ambio* 38, no. 6 (September 2009): 294.

7 **fifty-four billion pounds:** The global fisheries marine catch for 2014 was reported as 81.5 million metric tons by the Food and Agriculture Organization (FAO) of the United Nations. Forage fish, including anchovies and krill, are the generally smaller prey fish that sustain the marine food web and are estimated to comprise approximately 30 percent of the total global marine catch. Thirty percent of the total is 24.5 million metric tons, which in pounds equals 54 billion pounds of fish. Most of that catch is used in reduction industries for producing feed, fertilizer, and dietary supplements. For more information on forage fish, see E. Pikitch et al., *Little Fish, Big Impact: Managing a Crucial Link in Ocean Food Webs* (Washington, DC: Lenfest Ocean Program, 2012).

8 **Americans manage to eat only:** United States seafood consumption has hovered between twelve to fifteen pounds for the last decade. The most recent numbers show a slight increase. "Americans Added Nearly 1 Pound of Seafood to Their Diet in 2015," National Oceanic and Atmospheric Association, News and Features, October 26, 2016, www.noaa.gov/media-release/americans -added-nearly-1-pound-of-seafood-to-their-diet-in-2015.

8 **pounds of land food meat:** "Per Capita Consumption of Poultry and Livestock 1965 to 2018, Estimated in Pounds," National Chicken Council, www.nationalchickencouncil.org/about -the-industry/statistics/per-capita-consumption-of-poultry-and-livestock-1965-to-estimated -2012-in-pounds/.

CHAPTER ONE: ALGAE'S TOOLS

12 **Most relevant to the present:** This statement and much of the phytoplankton biochemical history and facts that follow are from a personal interview with Dr. Gary Wikfors conducted on June 22, 2017. Dr. Wikfors is a research fisheries biologist and also the chief of aquaculture sustainability and lab director of NOAA's Milford Laboratory in Connecticut. His own research as well as research of the NOAA lab in general focuses on shellfish aquaculture, which necessarily includes finding and testing the most efficient and nutritious food for bivalves—marine phytoplankton or microalgae. For more information on Wikfors's research, publications, and expertise, see his page on the Fisheries Service website: www.nefsc.noaa.gov/nefsc/Milford/staff/wikfors.html.

12 **oxygen-producing photosynthesis:** Cyanobacteria were the first organisms to be able to photosynthesize oxygen from visible light—a big step toward expanding life on earth. However, a half billion years before that, photosynthesis first appeared in earlier bacteria as a way to convert near-infrared light energy into sulfur-based compounds. See N. Y. Kiang, "The Color of Plants on Other Worlds," *Scientific American* 298 (2008): 48–55, and Becky Oskin, "When Did Earth's First Whiffs of Oxygen Emerge?," *Live Science*, March 23, 2014, www.livescience.com /44308-first-oxygen-breathers-on-earth.html.

13 **"rolls off the tongue easily":** Ralph Holman as quoted in Susan Allport, *The Queen of Fats: Why Omega-3s Were Removed from the Western Diet and What We Can Do to Replace Them* (Los Angeles and Berkeley: University of California Press, 2006), 43. The book is an excellent, thorough study of the research history and biochemistry of omega-3 fatty acids.

14 **The trillions upon trillions:** I was first introduced to this startling fact by Rowan Jacobson's excellent account of the 2010 Gulf oil spill: Rowan Jacobsen, *Shadows on the Gulf: A Journey Through Our Last Great Wetland* (New York: Bloomsbury USA, 2011).

15 **omega-6 fatty acids:** I. Lang et al., "Fatty Acid Profiles and Their Distribution Patterns in Microalgae: A Comprehensive Analysis of More Than 2000 Strains from the SAG Culture Collection," *BMC Plant Biology* 11 (2011): 124. This study of microalgae offers distinctions between chromophytes and chlorophytes on the level of phylum or class ranking based on the proportions of different fatty acids in their composition.

16 **This adaptation helped the dinoflagellates:** The early dinoflagellate eye is described in the Canadian Institute for Advanced Research, "Human-like 'Eye' in Single-Celled Plankton:

Mitochondria, Plastids Evolved Together," *ScienceDaily*, July 1, 2015, www.sciencedaily.com /releases/2015/07/150701133348.htm. For more information on dinoflagellates, including that preliminary eye, see Mona Hoppenrath and Juan F. Saldarriaga, "Dinoflagellates," Tree of Life web project, http://tolweb.org/Dinoflagellates/2445.

16 **concentrated in the red muscle:** There are two parts to explaining this statement. First, lipids are more concentrated in the red (slow twitch or tonic) muscle tissue in fish than the white (fast twitch) muscle tissue. See table in D. Houlihan, T. Boujard, and M. Jobling, eds., *Food Intake in Fish* (Oxford: Blackwell Science Ltd., 2001), 360. Second, the lipids in the muscles of fish have high concentrations of omega-3 fatty acids. For a breakdown of lipids in the tissues of fish, see J. M. Njinkoué et al., "Lipids and Fatty Acids in Muscle, Liver and Skin of Three Edible Fish from the Senegalese Coast: *Sardinella maderensis*, *Sardinella aurita* and *Cephalopholis taeniops*," *Comparative Biochemistry and Physiology Part B: Biochemistry and Molecular Biology* 131, no. 3 (March 2002): 395–402.

18 **"the negative phosphate groups":** Allport, *The Queen of Fats*, 96.

18 **"providing room for enzymes":** Ibid., 126.

18 **"will likely speed up":** A. J. Hulbert, "The Links Between Membrane Composition, Metabolic Rate and Lifespan," *Comparative Biochemistry and Physiology Part A: Molecular and Integrative Physiology* 150, no. 2 (June 2008): 196–203.

18 **what are called ion channels:** J. H. Langdon, "Has an Aquatic Diet Been Necessary for Hominid Brain Evolution and Functional Development?," *British Journal of Nutrition* 96 (2006): 7–17.

18 **the photoreceptors of:** John Paul SanGiovanni and Emily Y. Chew, "The Role of Omega-3 Long Chain Polyunsaturated Fatty Acids in Health and Disease of the Retina," *Progress in Retinal and Eye Research* 24, no. 1 (January 2005): 87–138.

19 **in concert with the eye:** The debate around which came first, the brain or the eye, is a persistent one that bothered Darwin himself. The high degree of complexity required for an organ to actually grant sight makes independent, gradual evolution of the eye seem highly unlikely. But when researchers at the University of Mainz in Germany examined early photoreceptors in a marine worm (*Platynereis dumerilii*) that lived up to six hundred million years ago, they found rod- and conelike structures similar to those of the human eye. On closer inspection they concluded that "two types of light-sensitive cells existed in our early animal ancestors: rhabdomeric and ciliary. In most animals, rhabdomeric cells became part of the eyes, and ciliary cells remained embedded in the brain. But the evolution of the human eye is peculiar—it is the ciliary cells that were recruited for vision which eventually gave rise to the rods and cones of the retina." Thus it seems plausible that the brain and the eye coevolved but that early incarnations of both had photoreceptivity as part of their inner chemical workings. European Molecular Biology Laboratory, "Darwin's Greatest Challenge Tackled: The Mystery of Eye Evolution," *ScienceDaily*, November 1, 2004, www.sciencedaily.com/releases/2004/10/041030215105.htm.

19 **a physician named Michael Crawford:** For a more complete history of Dr. Crawford's work, see Allport, *The Queen of Fats*, 87–95. My summaries of his research refer to his publications: M. A. Crawford and A. J. Sinclair, "Nutritional Influences in the Evolution of Mammalian Brain," in *Lipids, Malnutrition and the Developing Brain*, K. Elliot and J. Knight, eds. (Amsterdam: Elsevier, 1972), 267–92, and M. Crawford and D. Marsh, *The Driving Force: Food Evolution and the Future* (New York: Harper & Row, 1989).

20 **as few as two thousand:** Dr. David Whitehouse, "When Humans Faced Extinction," BBC News, June 9, 2003, http://news.bbc.co.uk/2/hi/science/nature/2975862.stm. For the original study see L. A. Zhivotovsky, N. A. Rosenberg, and M. W. Feldman, "Features of Evolution and Expansion of Modern Humans, Inferred from Genome-wide Microsatellite Markers," *American Journal of Human Genetics* 72, no. 5 (May 2003): 1171–86.

21 **they were sated:** This fictional scene was inspired by readings in Rowan Jacobsen, *The Living Shore: Rediscovering a Lost World* (New York: Bloomsbury USA, 2009).

21 **aquatic ape hypothesis:** Introduced to me by Erin Wayman, "A New Aquatic Ape Theory," Smithsonian.com, April 16, 2012, www.smithsonianmag.com/science-nature/a-new-aquatic -ape-theory-67868308/, which is based on the paper by R. Wrangham et al., "Shallow-Water Habitats as Sources of Fallback Foods for Hominids," *American Journal of Physical Anthropology* 140, no. 4 (December 2009): 630–42.

21 **"be considered to be unsupported":** Langdon, "Has an Aquatic Diet Been Necessary for Hominid Brain Evolution and Functional Development?," 7–17

22 **land plants do not contain:** J. T. Brenna, "Efficiency of Conversion of Alpha-Linolenic Acid to Long Chain n-3 Fatty Acids in Man," *Current Opinion in Clinical Nutrition and Metabolic Care* 5, no. 2 (March 2002): 127–32.

22 **a "cognitive revolution" took place:** Yuval Noah Harari, *Sapiens: A Brief History of Humankind* (London: Vintage Books, 2011): 23–25.

22 **In 2007 the remnants:** C. W. Marean, "Pinnacle Point Cave 13B (Western Cape Province, South Africa) in Context: The Cape Floral Kingdom, Shellfish, and Modern Human Origins," *Journal of Human Evolution* 59, no. 3–4 (September–October 2010): 425–43.

23 **huge shell piles:** Jon M. Erlandson writes in a 2013 issue of *Anthropocene* "Evidence for aquatic foraging, fishing, and scavenging by hominids dates back at least two million years, but aquatic resource use intensified with the appearance of *Homo sapiens*. The development of new fishing and seafaring technologies contributed to population growth and the spread of humans around the world. . . . After global sea level rise slowed eight-thousand years ago, a proliferation of shell middens formed an increasingly prominent stratigraphic signature for identifying and defining an Anthropocene Epoch." Jon Erlandson, "Shell Middens and Other Anthropogenic Soils as Global Stratigraphic Signatures of the Anthropocene," *Anthropocene* 4 (2013): 24–32.

23 **six centers around the world:** My brief overview of human history from hunter-gatherers to agriculture and specifically the six original centers of Neolithic agriculture can be found in M. Mazoyer and L. Roudart, *A History of World Agriculture: From the Neolithic Age to the Current Crisis* (New York: Monthly Review Press, 2006), 75.

CHAPTER TWO: THE SEA BETWEEN THE LANDS

26 **over a hundred years old:** Alan Maisel, "In One Italian Village, Nearly 300 Residents Are Over 100 Years Old," interview with Kelly McEvers and Audie Cornish, *All Things Considered*, NPR, March 30, 2016, audio, 2:29, www.npr.org/2016/03/30/472442367/in-one-italian-village-nearly-300-residents-are-over-100-years-old. A follow-up interview with the author took place on April 13, 2016.

30 **The first of these inquiries:** Allbaugh's research is summarized in Marion Nestle, "Mediterranean Diets: Historical and Research Overview," *American Journal of Clinical Nutrition* 61, no. 6 (Supplement) (July 1995): 1313S–20S.

31 **the Mediterranean island plots:** Mazoyer and Roudart, *A History of World Agriculture*, 447.

31 **"hungry most of the time":** Nestle, "Mediterranean Diets," 1315S.

33 **Keys and his biochemist wife:** For more detailed information on the history of Ancel Keys's original study and the subsequent research and publications, see 7 Countries Study website, www.sevencountriesstudy.com/about-the-study/.

34 **literally plugging up the works:** Allport, *The Queen of Fats*, 50–51.

34 **she began an analysis:** The history and opinions of Dr. Artemis Simopoulos are sourced from a personal interview with the author, March 17, 2016, Allport's *The Queen of Fats*, and Simopoulos's extensive publications. Some studies I explicitly reference include: A. P. Simopoulos and N. Salem Jr., "Purslane: A Terrestrial Source of Omega-3 Fatty Acids," *New England Journal of Medicine* 315, no. 13 (1986): 833; A. P. Simopoulos and N. Salem Jr., "N-3 Fatty Acids in Eggs from Range-Fed Greek Chickens," letter to the editor, *New England Journal of Medicine* 321 (1989): 1412; and A. P. Simopoulos, "Summary of the Conference on the Health Effects of Polyunsaturated Fatty Acids in Seafoods," *Journal of Nutrition* 116, no. 12 (January 1987): 2350–54.

36 **"the largest single change":** Captain Joseph Hibbeln, MD, interview with the author, May 23, 2017. Dr. Hibbeln is a clinical investigator and acting chief of the Laboratory of Membrane Biochemistry and Biophysics; Section of Nutritional Neuroscience at NIAAA at the National Institutes of Health.

36 **Inflammation has been implicated:** Jerome Groopman, "Inflamed: The Debate over the Latest Cure-All Craze," *The New Yorker*, November 30, 2015, www.newyorker.com/magazine/2015/11/30/inflamed.

37 **markedly different chemical directions:** Allport, *The Queen of Fats*, 97–102, specifically referencing Dr. William Lands's work on deciphering the different sources and behaviors of eicosanoids, including prostaglandins.

37 **enzymes will act upon:** The enzymes that metabolize the fatty acids treat omega-3s and omega-6s very similarly, almost identically, so they respond to the one in higher abundance, which

impairs the metabolism of the other. The competition between omega-3 and omega-6 for enzymatic attention was described "much like sibling rivalry" by the biochemist William Lands in an interview with the author, May 17, 2017.

38 ratio of about one-to-one: A. P. Simopoulos, "The Importance of the Ratio of Omega-6/Omega-3 Essential Fatty Acids," *Biomedicine and Pharmacotherapy* 56 (2002): 365–79.

39 lowering your risk: This statement and the following defense of Keys's work are from Dr. Walter Willett, personal interview with the author, August 14, 2017.

39 "the prevailing allegations are false": Dr. Katz's quote is from "True Health Initiative Releases White Paper on Seven Countries Study, Work of Ancel Keys," Cision PRWeb, November 9, 2017, www.prweb.com/releases/2017/08/prweb14557703.htm. And for the full white paper: K. D. Pett et al., "Ancel Keys and the Seven Countries Study: An Evidence-Based Response to Revisionist Histories," commissioned by the True Health Initiative, August 1, 2017, www.truehealthinitiative .org/wordpress/wp-content/uploads/2017/07/SCS-White-Paper.THI_.8-1-17.pdf.

41 the Paleo Diet: Dr. Loren Cordain is the founder of the Paleo Diet concept and author of numerous books on the topic, including the original, *The Paleo Diet*. The diet is based on the premise that eating foods that mimic the food groups of our preagricultural hunter-gatherer ancestors will help us optimize our health, minimize our risk of chronic disease, and lose weight. For more information see http://thepaleodiet.com/. Cordain readily acknowledges many influences in conceiving of a modern Paleo Diet. Most important to him was the work of Boyd Eaton, in particular S. Boyd Eaton and Melvin Konner, "Paleolithic Nutrition—A Consideration of Its Nature and Current Implications," *New England Journal of Medicine* 312 (January 1985): 283–89.

41 "without any one predominating": Hippocrates, "The Art of Medicine in Former Times. Section I—Treatise IV," *The Writings of Hippocrates and Galen*, John Redman Coxe, ed. and trans. (Philadelphia: Lindsay & Blakiston, 1846), 65.

43 "It is best to take": Reay Tannahill, *Food in History* (New York: Three Rivers Press, 1973), 83. As cited in an excellent thesis about the history of anchovies, salted fish, and fish sauce: Jill Santopietro, "Menaica Anchovies" (master's thesis, Boston University, 2014), 13.

44 major fish works were established: There is debate within the classics community about whether garum can be traced to Phoenicia. The strongest evidence is the consistent presence of salteries from Phoenician times on through Roman occupation. Extensive fish salting works that also produced garum can be found along the Spanish coast that date to the eighth century BCE. Founded by Phoenicians, they were expanded upon by Romans, where they produced garum into the imperial era. A description of the salteries and fish processing sites of Spain can be found in Darío Bernal Casasola, "Garum in Context: New Times, Same Topics in the Post-Ponsichian Era," in *The Inland Seas: Towards an Ecohistory of the Mediterranean and Black Sea*, T. Bekker-Nielsen and R. Gertwagen, eds. (Stuttgart: Franz Steiner Verlag, 2016), 187–214.

46 Iowa for the ancients: Mazoyer and Roudart, *A History of World Agriculture*, 149, 169, 246.

46 "fish were funny": Nicholas Purcell, "Eating Fish: The Paradoxes of Seafood," in *Food in Antiquity*, J. Wilkins, D. Harvey, and M. Dobson, eds. (Exeter, UK: Exeter University Press, 1995), 141–42.

46 "closest to human flesh": In an email to the author on April 22, 2016, Dr. John Wilkins wrote "You will see that Galen treats fish as less nourishing than meat, but finds big health benefits in grey mullet, sea bass and red mullet, which is the most nourishing fish because, he says, its flesh is closest to human flesh and needs least effort by the body to assimilate it. His idea of nourishment is close to ours of calorific value—what gives us energy and strength—and other properties that we think of as nutritious (vitamins, minerals, proteins etc.) he classifies as pharmacological."

47 Egyptian mummies were well salted: Tannahill, *Food in History*, 54. As cited by Santopietro, "Menaica Anchovies," 9.

47 re-created the process: Callum Roberts, *The Ocean of Life: The Fate of Man and the Sea* (New York: Penguin, 2012), 38.

47 An agronomist called Columella: Thomas H. Corcoran, "Roman Fish Sauces," *Classical Journal* 58, no. 5 (February 1963): 207. As cited by Santopietro, "Menaica Anchovies," 15.

48 much wider variety of ills: Mark Kurlansky, *Salt: A World History* (New York: Penguin, 2003), 71.

48 Garum also carried with it a promise: It is a notable coincidence that after brain cells, sperm cells have the highest amount of DHA omega-3 fatty acids, Allport, *The Queen of Fats*, 12.

48 Martial praises his friend Flaccus: Robert I. Curtis, "In Defense of Garum," *Classical Journal* 78, no. 3 (February–March 1983): 232.

48 **the cold reaches of Vindolanda:** Robert I. Curtis, "'Negotiatores Allecarii' and the Herring," *Phoenix* 38, no. 2 (Summer 1984): 151.

48 **In Apicius's *De re coquinaria*:** P. M. Zaret, "Liquamen and Other Fish Sauces," *Repast* 20, no. 4 (Fall 2004): 3. As cited in Santopietro, "Menaica Anchovies," 11.

48 **more profitably, a garum maker:** Purcell, "Eating Fish," 142.

49 **"the factory of Umbricus Agathopus":** Robert I. Curtis, "A Personalized Floor Mosaic from Pompeii," *American Journal of Archaeology* 88, no. 4 (October 1984), 564.

49 **cooked than to raw meat:** Peter F. Anson, *Fishermen and Fishing Ways*, facsimile of 1932 edition (Darlington, UK: EP Publishing Ltd, 1975), 30.

49 **The fish, hypnotized:** Anson, *Fishermen and Fishing Ways*, 31.

50 **Grudgingly, the sea's various nations:** András G. Inotai, cabinet member of the European Commissioner for Environment, Maritime Affairs and Fisheries, email to the author, April 5, 2016. A comprehensive study of the Mediterranean fisheries presented in 2016 found that only 5 percent of the exploited fish stocks in the area were fished sustainably. Many commercially important fish had mortality rates three to six times higher than the suggested maximum sustainable yield. Specific to sardines and anchovies, there were no catch limits. Minimum catch sizes and regulations regarding net mesh size and the distance that fishing can take place from the coast are in existence. Emergency measures to reduce fishing pressure as a precaution were put into place in 2014 and 2015 but have had little effect. Issues like these prompted Karmenu Vella, the European commissioner for Environment, Maritime Affairs and Fisheries, to include in the email, "The Commission has put the issue of the overexploitation of Mediterranean stocks high on the political agenda."

53 **The device was dropped:** Roberts, *The Ocean of Life*, 36.

53 **cycles of wind and weather:** Emily Farr, "Reading the Sea," *Currents and Tidings from Catania*, Pasta Madre Paradigm, June 10, 2016, http://pastamadreparadigm.com/features/2016/6/10 /currents-and-tidings-from-catania. Farr conducted interviews with fishermen throughout Italy to gauge the effect of environmental change. In "Reading the Sea" she interviewed Gaetano Urzì, the president of the fishers' cooperative in the Gulf of Catania, Sicily, who talked about how the seasonal weather had become unpredictable. See also Farr's master's thesis, "'*Non è come prima*': Observations of Climate Change by Small-Scale Coastal Fishers in Italy and the Role of Fishers' Knowledge," University of Gastronomic Sciences, 2016. For an overview of potential changes in the Mediterranean due to climate change, see F. Giorgi and P. Lionello, "Climate Change Projections for the Mediterranean Region," *Global and Planetary Change* 63 (2008): 90–104.

53 **But more disturbing:** Edward H. Allison et al., "Final Technical Report: Effects of Climate Change on the Sustainability of Capture and Enhancement Fisheries Important to the Poor: Analysis of the Vulnerability and Adaptability of Fisherfolk Living in Poverty," *Fisheries Management Science Programme: Department for International Development*, Project No. R4778J (2005).

54 **"Formerly he would look":** Farr, "*Non è come prima*," 15.

56 **the Mediterranean can no longer:** This is as true on land as it is on sea. In 2017 the Mediterranean olive crop was afflicted with the worst drought and hottest conditions in memory. Somini Sengupta, "How Climate Change Is Playing Havoc with Olive Oil (and Farmers)," *The New York Times*, October 24, 2017, www.nytimes.com/2017/10/24/climate/olive-oil.html?_r=0.

CHAPTER THREE: THE SUMMIT OF SUPPLEMENTISM

57 **half of all patients:** The physician in question here is Dariush Mozaffarian, dean of the Gerald J. and Dorothy R. Friedman School of Nutrition Science and Policy at Tufts University. Roughly 610,000 Americans die of heart disease annually ("Heart Disease Facts," Centers for Disease Control and Prevention, www.cdc.gov/heartdisease/facts.htm). Of those mortalities, 325,000 are attributed to sudden cardiac death, the most common form of natural death in the United States. "Sudden Cardiac Death (Sudden Cardiac Arrest)," Cleveland Clinic, https://my .clevelandclinic.org/health/articles/sudden-cardiac-death.

58 **Forrest Gump molecule:** Forrest Gump, the eponymous character of the 1986 novel by Winston Groom and 1994 film adaptation by Robert Zemeckis, manages through three decades of American life to stumble into the center of major trends from the hippie protests of the 1960s through the running craze of the 1970s on into the AIDS crisis of the 1980s. Winston Groom, *Forrest Gump* (New York: Doubleday, 1986).

58 **$15 billion annually:** It is hard to pin down exactly how much the omega-3 market is worth. The confusion arises in the value of fish oil supplements versus the value for supplemented products like infant formula, whose value is based only partially on omega-3s and partially to the overall contents of a given product. GOED in some instances estimates the market value of all omega-3 products to be $30 billion: "GOED: Omega-3 Finished Products Market Worth $31.4 Billion for 2015," *Nutraceuticals World,* June 22, 2016, www.nutraceuticalsworld.com/issues/2016-09/view _breaking-news/goed-omega-3-finished-products-market-worth-314-billion-for-2015/.   Isaac Berzin, a maker of algae-based omega-3, puts the valuation at closer to $15 billion: Isaac Berzin, interview with the author, July 16, 2016. Supplements in pill form, meanwhile, seem to be worth between $3 and $4 billion according to Dr. Enrico Bachis, the Market Research Director for IFFO (an international trade association that represents the fishmeal and fish oil industries).

59 **omega-3 supplementation to prostate cancer:** A 2013 controversial case-cohort study by Theodore M. Brasky and colleagues found that high levels of omega-3 increased the risk of developing prostate cancer by 44 percent. T. M. Brasky et al., "Plasma Phospholipid Fatty Acids and Prostate Cancer Risk in the SELECT Trial," *Journal of the National Cancer Institute* 105 (2013): 1132–41.

59 **"was not associated with":** E. C. Rizos et al., "Association Between Omega-3 Fatty Acid Supplementation and Risk of Major Cardiovascular Disease Events." It was later resupported by another *JAMA* meta-analysis study: A. Grey and M. Bolland, "Clinical Trial Evidence and Use of Fish Oil Supplements," *JAMA Internal Medicine* 174, no. 3 (2014): 460–62.

59 **"could be considered over now":** Dr. Gianni Tognoni's quote is from A. O'Connor, "Fish Oil Claims Not Supported by Research," *The New York Times,* March 30, 2015, https://well.blogs.ny times.com/2015/03/30/fish-oil-claims-not-supported-by-research/?mcubz=1&_r=1. The study the article referenced: Risk and Prevention Study Collaborative Group, M. C. Roncaglioni et al., "N-3 Fatty Acids in Patients with Multiple Cardiovascular Risk Factors," *New England Journal of Medicine* 368, no. 19 (May 9, 2013): 1800–1808.

60 **different *Frontline* film:** The director and producer were Neil Docherty and *Frontline*'s creator, David Fanning. The *Frontline* documentary that I anchored and cowrote is Paul Greenberg, "The Fish on My Plate," *Frontline,* PBS, season 34, episode 15, April 25, 2017, film, 1:26:46, www.pbs.org/video/the-fish-on-my-plate-nsxhez/.

60 **A rotten fish oil capsule:** "Supplements and Safety," *Frontline,* PBS, season 34, episode 3, January 19, 2016, film, 54:11, www.pbs.org/video/frontline-supplements-and-safety/.

60 **"every single meta-analysis":** Ismail, "What *Frontline* Didn't Say About Omega-3s."

61 **"We all know":** Adam Ismail, "Welcome," filmed at the GOED Exchange 2016 Conference, Tenerife, Canary Islands. Uploaded March 2, 2016, video, 37:06, www.youtube.com/watch?v= WCqZjOVlgB8&list=PLHYxROoZNvQyKkhGq5d2_u_E890w8USXC&index=29.

61 **non-randomized controlled trials:** Michelle Wiest, "The Value of Non-RCT Research," GOED Exchange 2016 Conference Program, February 4, 2016, https://custom.cvent.com /2CB4EE6B04744A398EB918810001D792/files/event/A238FEDFFF374F3FB1E 3D80A9A5A39D3/044000ec7425436ebdbd17280c688265.pdf.

61 **promised to reveal:** "The Omega-3 Trust Paradox," GOED Exchange 2016 Conference Program, February 2, 2016, https://custom.cvent.com/2CB4EE6B04744A398EB918810001D792 /files/event/A238FEDFFF374F3FB1E3D80A9A5A39D3/044000ec7425436ebdbd172 80c688265.pdf.

61 **campaign to eliminate trans fats:** According to Dyerberg "Denmark was the first nation to implement—in 2004—a trans fat ban against the use of industrially produced trans fatty acids (IPTFA), setting an upper limit of 2 percent of IPTFA in fat used for human food. This has since been copied in several countries (Norway, Iceland, Switzerland, Canada, etc.). Together with my colleagues Dr. Stender and Dr. Astrup we were the leading scientists on the Danish Nutritional Board, which spearheaded the pressure on the government to legislate against trans fat." Email from Jørn Dyerberg, November 23, 2017.

63 **"let's do whatever we can!":** Jørn Dyerberg, interviews with the author, February 2, 2016, and May 11, 2016. To read the original paper on the plasma lipids of Eskimos, see H. O. Bang, J. Dyerberg, and A. B. Nielsen, "Plasma Lipid and Lipoprotein Pattern in Greenlandic West-Coast Eskimos," *Lancet* 297, no. 7710 (June 1971): 1143–46.

64 **transported to gonads:** Eric Schultz, interview with the author, June 8, 2016, and email to the author, November 13, 2017. Dr. Schultz is an associate professor at the Department of Ecology and Evolutionary Biology, University of Connecticut.

64 **Somewhere around 700 CE:** "History of Cod Liver Oil," Rosita, http://evclo.com/history/.

65 **now known as rickets:** For the history of the diagnosis and early treatments of rickets, see Jeffrey L. H. O'Riordan and Olva L. M. Bijvoet, "Rickets Before the Discovery of Vitamin D," *BoneKEy Reports* 3, no. 478 (January 8, 2014): 1–6, www.nature.com/bonekeyreports/2014 /140108/bonekey2013212/full/bonekey2013212.html.

65 **"laundry put out to dry":** Quoted from O'Riordan and Bijvoet, "Rickets Before the Discovery of Vitamin D," 4, in reference to Claire Tomalin, *Samuel Pepys: The Unequalled Self* (London: Penguin, 2002).

66 **effective in curing rickets:** O'Riordan and Bijvoet, "Rickets Before the Discovery of Vitamin D," 5.

66 **churned out five thousand barrels:** "Möller's Brand History," Möllers Omega-3, 2017, www .mollersomega3.com/about-mollers/mollers-brand-history/.

67 **Vitamin D helps the gut:** "Vitamin D: Fact Sheet for Consumers," National Institutes of Health, https://ods.od.nih.gov/factsheets/VitaminD-Consumer/, and "Vitamin A: Fact Sheet for Consumers," National Institutes of Health, https://ods.od.nih.gov/factsheets/VitaminA-Consumer/.

67 **"dietary enrichment with EPA":** This quote is the concluding sentence of the abstract in the landmark paper published by Dyerberg, Bang, and their collaborators: J. Dyerberg et al., "Eicosapentaenoic Acid and Prevention of Thrombosis and Atherosclerosis?," *Lancet* 2, no. 8081 (July 15, 1978): 117–19.

67 **"Association studies will tell you":** Martina Pavlicova, email to the author, November 13, 2017. Dr. Pavlicova is an associate professor of biostatistics at Columbia University.

68 **recovered from scurvy:** See James Lind, *Treatise of the Scurvy: In Three Parts* (Edinburgh: Sands, Murray, & Cochran, 1753), 191–96, www.jameslindlibrary.org/lind-j-1753/ for details of Lind's scurvy trials as well as other writings on the evolution of clinical trials.

69 **Placebos were famously administered:** Robert Jütte, "The Early History of the Placebo," *Complementary Therapies in Medicine* 21, no. 2 (April 2013): 94–97.

69 **"a real psychotherapeutic effect":** Quote on Graves's research by M. D. Yapko, *Trancework: An Introduction to the Practice of Clinical Hypnosis* (New York: Routledge, 2012), 123. And the original 1920 paper with Graves's thoughts on placebos: T. C. Graves, "Commentary on a Case of Hystero-epilepsy with Delayed Puberty: Treated with Testicular Extract," *Lancet* 196 (1920): 1134–35.

70 **the gold standard:** One of the physicians participating in the streptomycin study wrote about his experience and the legacy of the double-blind randomized trial in J. Crofton, "The MRC Randomized Trial of Streptomycin and Its Legacy: A View from the Clinical Front Line," *Journal of the Royal Society of Medicine* 99, no. 10 (October 2006): 531–34.

70 **Bang and Dyerberg's discoveries:** Published in 1989, the DART trial was the first randomized controlled trial to test Bang and Dyerberg's hypothesis that fish oils could protect against coronary heart disease. Results showed a reduction in all-cause mortality over two years in men with a recent history of myocardial infarction after taking 300 grams of oily fish per week or fish oil supplements with equivalent levels of omega-3 fatty acids. The DART trial findings were then confirmed by the GISSI-Prevenzione trial. M. L. Burr et al., "Effects of Changes in Fat, Fish, and Fibre Intakes on Death and Reinfarction: Diet and Reinfarction Trial," *Lancet* 334, no. 8666 (September 30, 1989): 757–61; and Stone, "The GISSI–Prevenzione Trial on Fish Oil and Vitamin E Supplementation in Myocardial Infarction Survivors."

70 **reducing cardiovascular disease:** Dyerberg and Bang et al., "Eicosapentaenoic Acid and Prevention of Thrombosis and Atherosclerosis?" Note the question mark at the end of the paper's title.

71 **something now called a ketogenic diet:** The ketogenic mode of eating has heavily influenced popular weight loss programs like the South Beach Diet and the Whole 30. It was initially used, however, to treat epilepsy and later revived in popular food culture when the Hollywood producer Jill Abrahams successfully used it to treat her epileptic son. A made-for-TV movie adapted from the story, called *First Do No Harm* and starring Meryl Streep, drove home the point.

72 **multimillion-dollar operation:** Aker BioMarine's investment in krill continues to grow apace, with the company in 2017 commissioning the construction of a 1 billion NOK ($122 million USD) krill fishing vessel. "Building New Krill Vessel," Aker BioMarine, April 14, 2017, www .akerbiomarine.com/news/aker-biomarine-to-build-new-krill-vessel.

72 **chance of a fishy burp:** Hallvard Muri, personal interview with the author, September 23, 2015. Muri is the CEO of AKVA group ASA of global aquaculture technology and services. Previously he was the CEO of Aker BioMarine for over six years.

73 **"At first people":** Sonja Connor, interview with the author, June 17, 2013.

74 **"the consumption of fish":** "Letter Regarding Dietary Supplement Health Claim for Omega-3 Fatty Acids and Coronary Heart Disease," U.S. Food and Drug Administration, Center for Food Safety and Applied Nutrition, Office of Nutritional Products, Labeling, and Dietary Supplements, Docket No. 91N-0103 (October 31, 2000), www.fda.gov/ohrms/dockets/dockets/95s0316/95s-0316-Rpt0272-38-Appendix-D-Reference-F-FDA-vol205.pdf.

74 **inflammation a "research priority":** Groopman, "Inflamed: The Debate over the Latest Cure-All Craze."

75 **government-required clinical trials:** Thirty-seven billion dollars per year in 2014 for the United States alone, according to the National Institutes of Health. "Multivitamin/mineral Supplements: Fact Sheet for Health Professionals," National Institutes of Health, https://ods.od.nih.gov/factsheets/MVMS-HealthProfessional/.

75 **traveling cowboy-huckster:** For the whole snake oil story, see Dan Hurley, *Natural Causes: Death, Lies and Politics in America's Vitamin and Herbal Supplement Industry* (New York: Crown, 2006), 23–26.

77 **Linus Pauling is credited:** Pauling's vitamin C obsession is detailed in Paul A. Offit, *Do You Believe in Magic? Vitamins, Supplements, and All Things Natural: A Look Behind the Curtain* (New York: HarperCollins, 2013), 51–62.

77 **the Proxmire Amendment:** Named after Senator William Proxmire of Wisconsin. For a good overview of vitamin and supplement regulation history in the United States, see W. S. Pray, "The FDA, Vitamins, and the Dietary Supplement Industry," *U.S. Pharmacist* 33, no. 10 (2008): 10–15.

77 **the most humiliating defeat:** P. A. Offit, "Don't Take Your Vitamins," *The New York Times*, June 8, 2013, www.nytimes.com/2013/06/09/opinion/sunday/dont-take-your-vitamins.html.

77 **Utah senator Orrin Hatch:** According to Dan Hurley's *Natural Causes* (as cited in Paul Offit's *Do You Believe in Magic?*, cited above), between 1989 and 1994, Hatch received $49,250 from HerbaLife International, $31,500 from MetaboLife, and $88,550 from Rexall Sundown, Nu Skin International, and Starlight International. Hatch also owned 35,621 shares of Pharmics, a Utah-based nutritional supplement company. Hurley, *Natural Causes*, 75–77.

77 **"a third hermaphroditic category":** Hurley, *Natural Causes*, as cited in Offit, *Do You Believe in Magic?*, 87.

78 **medical watchdog Peter Gøtzsche:** Peter C. Gøtzsche, "Why We Need Easy Access to All Data from All Clinical Trials and How to Accomplish It," *Trials* 12 (November 23, 2011): 249. Gøtzsche and his research collaborators were frequently cited in a review study that concluded, "Sponsorship of drug and device studies by the manufacturing company leads to more favorable results and conclusions than sponsorship by other sources. Our analyses suggest the existence of an industry bias that cannot be explained by standard 'risk of bias' assessments." A. Lundh et al., "Industry Sponsorship and Research Outcome (Review)," The Cochrane Collaboration, *The Cochrane Library* 7 (New York: John Wiley and Sons, 2013), 2, www.abc.net.au/catalyst/heartofthematter/download/Industrysponsorshiptaintsthescience.pdf.

79 **Taylor had been hired:** Judy Taylor, "The Omega-3 Trust Paradox," filmed at the GOED Exchange 2016 Conference, Tenerife, Canary Islands. Uploaded March 4, 2016, video, 30:39, https://www.youtube.com/watch?v=WCqZjOVlgB8&list=PLHYxROoZNvQyKkhGq5d2_u_E890w8USXC&index=29.

82 **handful of medical papyri:** As Michael North, curator of the National Library of Medicine's rare books collection within the library's History of Medicine Division, put it, "[The Edwin Smith Papyrus] is unlike most other medical papyri in that it is chiefly rational and does not usually bring the supernatural into the explanations or treatments for injuries." "An Ancient Medical Treasure at Your Fingertips," U.S. National Library of Medicine, NIH, last updated July 29, 2013, www.nlm.nih.gov/news/turn_page_egyptian.html. The full Edwin Smith papyrus can be found online at https://ceb.nlm.nih.gov/proj/ttp/flash/smith/smith.html.

83 **at *The New York Times*:** Alexander Star, email to the author, November 1, 2016. Mr. Star, formerly of *The New York Times Magazine*, is now a senior editor at Farrar, Straus & Giroux.

83 **a statistician named Michelle Wiest:** Michelle Wiest, "The Value of Non-RCT Research," filmed at the GOED Exchange 2016 Conference, Tenerife, Canary Islands. Uploaded March 2, 2016, video, 26:50, www.youtube.com/watch?v=RLOK0R2E_G8&list=PLHYxROoZNvQyKkhGq5d2_u_E890w8USXC&index=26.

84 **Fifty different fraudulent academic journals:** The actual Polish word for fraud is *oszust*—but the authors are clearly playing a semantic game here. From Alan Burdick, "'Paging Dr. Fraud': The

Fake Publishers That Are Ruining Science," *The New Yorker,* March 22, 2017, www.newyorker
.com/tech/elements/paging-dr-fraud-the-fake-publishers-that-are-ruining-science.

86 **when I asked Martina Pavlicova:** Martina Pavlicova, emails to the author, November 11–17, 2017. Dr. Pavlicova, at my request, reviewed Rizos et al. and conveyed her impressions to me over a weeklong correspondence.

87 **an overall 6 percent decrease:** G. C. Chen et al., "N-3 Long Chain Polyunsaturated Fatty Acids and Risk of All-Cause Mortality Among General Populations: A Meta-analysis," *Scientific Reports* 6, no. 28165 (June 16, 2016).

87 **Statins have a proven effect:** For an overview of studies done on the anti-inflammatory effects of mushrooms and statins, see E. A. Elsayedet al., "Mushrooms: A Potential Natural Source of Anti-inflammatory Compounds for Medical Applications," *Mediators of Inflammation* 2014, no. 805841 (November 23, 2014): 1–15.

88 **fatal coronary heart disease:** A recent study showed that individuals with omega-3 levels at 8 percent of blood lipid levels had a 30 percent reduced rate of fatal coronary heart disease compared with those whose omega-3 blood lipid levels were at 4 percent. William S. Harris, Liana Del Gobbo, and Nathan L. Tintle, "The Omega-3 Index and Relative Risk for Coronary Heart Disease Mortality: Estimation from 10 Cohort Studies," *Atherosclerosis* 262 (2017): 51–54.

89 **huge "megabucks" studies:** A summary of large-scale omega-3 trials under way as of this writing can be found in K. J. Bowen, W. S. Harris, and P. M. Kris-Etherton, "Omega-3 Fatty Acids and Cardiovascular Disease: Are There Benefits?," *Current Treatment Options in Cardiovascular Medicine* 18, no. 11 (2016): 69, www.ncbi.nlm.nih.gov/pmc/articles/PMC5067287/.

89 **25,874 participants for six years:** The study tested the possible health effects of both vitamin D and omega-3s with an emphasis on heart disease and cancer. In the end, no significant correlation was found between omega-3 supplementation and the risk of developing cancer. Heart disease results were more complicated. As the authors reported: "During the trial, 386 major cardiovascular disease events occurred among the 12,933 participants receiving omega-3 fatty acids, as compared with 419 such events among the 12,938 participants receiving placebo, an 8% reduction that was not significant. Upon closer examination, this result was due almost entirely to a reduction in heart attacks without a reduction in strokes. Specifically, the omega-3 fatty acid intervention lowered the risk of heart attack by 28% and the risk of fatal heart attack by 50% but had no benefit on stroke or cardiovascular deaths not related to heart disease." Curiously, the most significant finding occurred within the African American subgroup of the study, where "omega-3 fatty acid supplementation led to a 19% reduction in major cardiovascular events, including a 40% reduction in heart attack, as well as a trend toward a reduction in death from any cause." Supplementation further led "to a 77% reduction in heart attacks, and a benefit was observed regardless of level of fish intake." Nevertheless, the researchers concluded, "some of these findings may have been due to chance and should not be viewed as conclusive." The conclusions of the VITAL study can be found at https://www.vitalstudy.org/findings.html.

CHAPTER FOUR: THE REPUBLIC OF REDUCTIONISM

92 **rates of cardiovascular disease:** The Canadian cardiologist George Fodor examined Greenland health records and concluded it was "highly unlikely" that local health officials were able to record accurately incidences of cardiac death. As *Slate* later reported, "30 percent of people lived in settlements with no medical officer at all. This meant many death certificates were filled out by whoever was nearby, without a doctor ever seeing the body. Someone experiencing heart attack symptoms might not be close enough to a hospital to attempt a trip. Even if he did, the hospital might have limited equipment for diagnosis. And 20 percent of heart attacks cause sudden death." Elizabeth Preston, "The Fishy Origins of the Fish Oil Craze," *Slate,* August 3, 2014, www.slate .com/articles/health_and_science/medical_examiner/2014/08/does_fish_oil _prevent_heart_disease_original_danish_eskimo_diet_study_was.html.

92 **one in every four fish:** The one-in-four statistic reflects the fact that "a quarter of the world's commercially caught fish, 20 million tons of wild seafood, is directed away from our dinner plates every year, and instead is used for fishmeal production." This quote is taken from Clare Leschin-Hoar, "90 Percent of Fish We Use for Fishmeal Could Be Used to Feed Humans Instead," *The Salt,* NPR, February 13, 2017, www.npr.org/sections/thesalt/2017/02/13 /515057834/90-percent-of-fish-we-use-for-fishmeal-could-be-used-to-feed-humans-instead.

And the story is based on a scientific paper: T. Cashion et al., "Most Fish Destined for Fishmeal Production Are Food-Grade Fish," *Fish and Fisheries* 18 (2017): 837–44.

93 **Upwellings occur throughout the world:** A more detailed description of how upwellings work can be found in Roberts, *The Ocean of Life*, 70–75.

94 **If the anchoveta are removed:** A comprehensive discussion of the ecological role played by forage fish can be found in Pikitch et al., "Little Fish Big Impact," www.lenfestocean.org /~/media/legacy/lenfest/pdfs/littlefishbigimpact_revised_12june12.pdf?la=en.

94 **anchoveta go into lockdown:** For the specific cycle of El Niño (and La Niña) and the effect on Peruvian fisheries are see Becky Oskin, "What Is El Niño?," *Live Science*, August 20, 2015, www .livescience.com/3650-el-nino.html.

95 **another research vessel:** The annual Peruvian fishery has two seasons, the first generally in May through July, and the second in November through January. The break between the two seasons allows time for the anchovies to spawn. In 2015, the first fishing season occurred per usual as recorded in "Evaluation of the North-Center Stock of the Peruvian Anchoveta. Current Status and Management Recommendations for the First Fishing Season 2015," IMARPE (July 2015), 36. But in September of the same year, just before the second season was to begin IMARPE conducted a survey and found that due to ocean and weather conditions the spawning season had not restored the anchovy stock to the necessary minimum biomass. At that time IMARPE stated that no quota could be set for the second spawning season as documented in "Situation of the North-Central Stock of the Peruvian Anchoveta to September of 2015," IMARPE (September 2015), 36. After an additional survey was conducted in October, IMARPE declared numbers high enough to allow a second season, which began the second week of November 2015: "Supplementary Report on the Situation of the North-Central Stock of Peruvian Anchoveta in November 2015," IMARPE (November 2015), 10–11.

95 **counting and recounting:** Patricia Majluf relayed these impressions to me on camera for an interview I did with her for the PBS program *Frontline:* Greenberg, "The Fish on My Plate," www.pbs .org/video/the-fish-on-my-plate-nsxhez/.

97 **the last Inca king, Atahualpa:** John Hemming, *The Conquest of the Incas* (New York: Houghton Mifflin Harcourt, 1970), 49.

98 **the guano islands were ignored:** J. M. Jensen, "Who Shall Have the Desert? Origin of the Controversy over South American Nitrate Lands," *The Improvement Era* 25 (June 1922): 677–80.

98 **the soils of the Northern Hemisphere were giving out:** See D. Duffy, "The Guano Islands of Peru: The Once and Future Management of a Renewable Resource," *Birdlife Conservation Series* 1 (1994): 68–76.

99 **bones of the buffalo:** A. C. Isenberg, *The Destruction of the Bison* (Cambridge, MA: Cambridge University Press, 2000), 160–62.

99 **Alexander von Humboldt:** The many travels and discoveries of Alexander von Humboldt are vividly depicted in this superb biography: Andrea Wulf, *The Invention of Nature: Alexander Von Humboldt's New World* (New York: Alfred A. Knopf, 2015).

99 **" admiration of his famous personal narrative":** Ibid., 257.

100 **He quickly saw that the nitrogen:** G. T. Cushman, *Guano and the Opening of the Pacific World* (New York: Cambridge University Press, 2013), 28–29.

101 **Shells of the destroyed eggs:** Duffy, "The Guano Islands of Peru," 70.

101 **fish called menhaden:** My accounts of the menhaden industry are drawn primarily from H. Bruce Franklin, *The Most Important Fish in the Sea: Menhaden and America* (Washington, DC: Island Press, 2009), and W. Jeffrey Bolster, *The Mortal Sea: Fishing the Atlantic in the Age of Sail* (Cambridge, MA: Harvard University Press, 2012).

102 **particularly good as fertilizer:** Franklin, *The Most Important Fish in the Sea*, 52.

102 **promise of $11 per barrel:** Bolster, *The Mortal Sea*, 125.

102 **along the Norwegian coastline:** Information about early Norwegian reduction fisheries is from Vegard Denstadli of the Norwegian feed manufacturer BioMar, emails to the author, October 31 and November 1, 2017.

103 **first offensive action:** Operation Claymore was a covert raid on the Lofoten Islands of Norway on March 4, 1941. A commando force landed at Stamsund and destroyed the Lofoten's Cod Boiling Plant. Factories were also destroyed at Henningsvær and Svolvær. In total, about 800,000 imperial gallons of fish oil were incinerated. *Journal of Military History* 73, no. 2 (April 2009): 471–95 | 10.1353/jmh.0.0285.

104 The American Heart Association: "The Skinny on Fats," American Heart Association, www .heart.org/HEARTORG/Conditions/Cholesterol/PreventionTreatmentofHighCholesterol /The-Skinny-on-Fats_UCM_305628_Article.jsp#.WgmttoZry7o.

104 the wholesale slaughter: The convergence of margarine, Norwegian independence, and whales is recounted in Ian B. Hart, *Whaling in the Falkland Islands Dependencies 1904–1931: A History of Shore and Bay-Based Whaling in the Antarctic* (Trowbridge, UK: Cromwell Press, 2006), 9–13.

105 led the most hardened whalers: D. Graham Burnett, *The Sounding of the Whale: Science and Cetaceans in the Twentieth Century* (Chicago: University of Chicago Press, 2012), 64–67.

106 15 and 32 percent: Hart, *Whaling in the Falkland Islands Dependencies 1904–1931,* 119.

106 Southern Hemisphere blue whales: Based on population estimates from the International Union for Conservation of Nature, "*Balaenoptera musculus* (Blue Whale)," The IUCN Red List of Threatened Species, www.iucnredlist.org/details/2477/0.

106 the British mathematician Colin Clark: Melanie Challenger, *On Extinction: How We Became Estranged from Nature* (Berkeley, CA: Counterpoint, 2012), 130.

107 great minds of the sea: For a table of whale products produced during this era see Hart, *Whaling in the Falkland Islands Dependencies 1904–1931,* 112.

107 Californians turned to something: My account of the California sardine fishery is drawn primarily from E. Ueber and A. MacCall, "The Rise and Fall of the California Sardine Empire," in *Climate Variability, Climate Change, and Fisheries,* Michael H. Glantz, ed. (Cambridge, MA: Cambridge University Press, 2005), 31–47.

108 California Department of Fish and Game: Ibid., 33–35.

110 In warmer temperatures: Elizabeth Grossman, "A Little Fish with Big Impact in Trouble on US West Coast," *Yale Environment 360,* June 18, 2015, http://e360.yale.edu/feature/a_little _fish_with_big_impact_in_trouble_on_us_west_coast/2887/.

110 moved to Peru: Ueber and MacCall, "The Rise and Fall of the California Sardine Empire," 43–44.

110 homeland of whale-based reductionism: Nils Kolle et al., *Fish, Coast and Communities: A History of Norway* (Bergen: Fagbokforlaget, 2017), 223.

114 from forty-five million birds: Claes Brundenius, "The Rise and Fall of the Peruvian Fishmeal Industry," *Instant Research on Peace and Violence* 3, no. 3 (1973): 149–58.

115 Now there are strict limits: Ibid., 156; and Humberto Speziani, the senior management adviser of TASA, one of Peru's largest fishing companies, interview with the author, March 21, 2016.

115 "If there's no human demand": Andrew Mallison, interview with the author, November 8, 2017.

117 weight of twelve hundred pounds: Michael Pollan, "Power Steer," *The New York Times Magazine,* March 31, 2002.

117 "If all of the crop": Dana Grunders, "Wasted: How America Is Losing Up to 40 Percent of Its Food from Farm to Fork to Landfill," Natural Resources Defense Council (NRDC) Issue Paper, August 2012, IP:12-06-B, www.nrdc.org/sites/default/files/wasted-food-IP.pdf.

117 a host of other amino acids: R. D. Miles and J. P. Jacob, "Fishmeal: Understanding Why This Feed Ingredient Is So Valuable in Poultry Diets," University of Florida, Institute of Food and Agricultural Sciences, document PS30, 1997, http://ufdcimages.uflib.ufl.edu/IR/00/00/42 /64/00001/PS04300.pdf.

117 American animal confinement: The early growth of U.S. CAFOs in the 1950s coincides nearly exactly with the Peruvian anchovy fishmeal production boom from 1957 to 1963. For a thorough investigation of the history and politics behind the development of the Peruvian fishery, see Kristin Wintersteen, "Fishing for Food and Fodder: The Transnational Environmental History of Humboldt Current Fisheries in Peru and Chile since 1945" (PhD dissertation, Duke University, 2011).

118 turned to anchoveta: This is a summary of the nationalization, then denationalization, of the fishery industry in Peru during and after Alvarado's presidency. The central government took full control after the fishery declined due to overfishing, debt, and an El Niño event. See "Peru Takes Over Declining Fisheries," *The New York Times,* May 9, 1973, www.nytimes.com /1973/05/09/archives/peru-takes-over-declining-fisheries-bad-weather-conditions-attempt. html. See also Wintersteen, "Fishing for Food and Fodder," for events during Alvarado's era.

118 the unknown growth factor: G. H. Arscott and G. F. Combs, "Unidentified Growth Factors Required by Chicks and Poults," *Poultry Science* 34, no. 4 (July 1955): 843–50.

118 Pregnant sows fed fishmeal: J. H. Cho and I. H. Kim, "Fish Meal—Nutritive Value," *Journal of Animal Physiology and Animal Nutrition* 95 (2011): 685–92.

118 meta-analysis of 196 papers: D. Średnicka-Tober et al., "Composition Differences Between Organic and Conventional Meat: A Systematic Literature Review and Meta-analysis," *British Journal of Nutrition* 115, no. 6 (March 28, 2016): 994–1011; D. Średnicka-Tober et. al., "Higher PUFA and n-3 PUFA, Conjugated Linoleic Acid, α-Tocopherol and Iron, but Lower Iodine and Selenium Concentrations in Organic Milk: A Systematic Literature Review and Meta- and Redundancy Analyses," *British Journal of Nutrition* 115, no. 6 (March 28, 2016): 1043–60.

119 68 percent of homes: "Pet Industry Market Size & Ownership Statistics," American Pet Products Association (APPA), www.americanpetproducts.org/press_industrytrends.asp.

119 "happy family life required pets": Katherine C. Grier, email to the author, July 7, 2016. Grier is, in addition to a pet industry scholar, a professor and the director of the Museum Studies Program at the University of Delaware. She published a history of human-animal relationships in America called *Pets in America: A History* (Chapel Hill: University of North Carolina Press, 2006).

119 The great maw of the renderers: Geoffrey S. Becker, "Animal Rendering: Economics and Policy," *Congressional Research Service (CRS) Report for Congress*, Order Code RS2 1771, updated March 17, 2004, http://nationalaglawcenter.org/wp-content/uploads/assets/crs /RS21771.pdf.

120 particularly high in taurine: A. R. Spitze et al., "Taurine Concentrations in Animal Feed Ingredients; Cooking Influences Taurine Content," *Journal of Animal Physiology and Animal Nutrition* 87 (2003): 251–62.

120 worth over $24 billion: The actual value for 2016 was $24.6 billion, with a prediction of $30 billion by 2022. "U.S. Pet Food Market Forecast at US $30 billion by 2022," Petfood Industry .com, January 6, 2017, www.petfoodindustry.com/articles/6224-us-pet-food-market-forecast-at -us30-billion-by-2022.

120 Chinese aquaculture has grown: China's growth as an aquaculture powerhouse is discussed in my book *American Catch: The Fight for Our Local Seafood* (New York: Penguin Press, 2014), 185–92.

121 China Fishery Group acquired Copeinca: For the back-and-forth of the Chinese involvement in Peruvian anchoveta, see Colin Post, "Distressed Chinese Firm to Sell Peru's Largest Fishery," *Peru Reports*, January 7, 2016, https://perureports.com/2016/01/07/distressed-chinese -firm-to-sell-perus-largest-fishery/; and Jason Smith, "Trustee Moves to Kick off China Fishery Sale; Cites 65 Interested Parties," *Undercurrent News*, July 28, 2017, www.undercurrentnews .com/2017/07/28/trustee-moves-to-kick-off-china-fishery-sale-cites-65-interested-parties/. Cooke Aquaculture's acquisition of Omega Protein is here: "Cooke Inks $500m Deal for Omega Protein," *Undercurrent News*, October 6, 2017, www.undercurrentnews.com/2017/10/06 /cooke-inks-deal-for-omega-protein/.

121 most low-carbon foods: R.W.R. Parker and P. H. Tyedmers, "Fuel Consumption of Global Fishing Fleets: Current Understanding and Knowledge Gaps," *Fish and Fisheries* 16, no. 4 (June 2014): 684–96.

122 talk about all this: My discussion with Mr. Speziani was filmed for a PBS *Frontline* special, and the present account condenses both the actual onscreen appearance of Mr. Speziani as well as the transcript made from the full interview by the *Frontline* producers. The completed *Frontline* documentary is "The Fish on My Plate," *Frontline*, PBS, season 34, episode 15, April 25, 2017; film, 1:26:46, www.pbs.org/video/the-fish on my plate-sxhez/.

123 "we didn't see the future": Mr. Speziani's quotation has been partially corrected to make the English phraseology more intelligible. The full quotation verbatim from the *Frontline* transcript is: "...definitely, definitely. Of course we are partially culprit, yes. Because we don't—we don't— the law is the Congress, the government executive, but it's—we didn't saw the future. We were more concerned—I don't know. If that was a mistake of the industry, yes. It was a mistake of the government, yes. Both. It's not only the government. We are truly—I don't know—it's a very good question. Yes and we—that needs to be changed and we can decide according to the market. You start developing a different market."

124 triglycerides sometimes go: This information was conveyed to me by Sandro Lane, a manufacturer of omega-3 supplements derived from salmon oil. As Lane put it to me in an email, "Omega-3 levels in crude fish oils vary greatly between harvest seasons, catch regions, and species of fish. This presents a problem if you are trying to meet a label specification on a dietary supplement. . . . How do you standardize the oil to reach an industry standard 18:12 level (18 percent EPA: 12

percent DHA) that they want to claim? You distill it. No fish naturally swims in the ocean with an 18:12 EPA DHA level. Those are manmade specifications that arise from refining." Lane then went on to explain that humans evolved consuming omega-3's in their natural triglyceride form. The ethyl ester form that many manufacturers employ is actually an alcohol and not a fat. The reformed triglycerides, Lane noted, are often marketed as similar to natural triglycerides Sandro Lane, email to author November 27, 2017.

125 **"So, you need to be":** Dave Matthews is quoted from his appearance on Greenberg, "The Fish on My Plate," www.pbs.org/wgbh/frontline/film/the-fish-on-my-plate/.

CHAPTER FIVE: HEARTLAND

128 **top ten sources of calories:** U.S. Department of Agriculture and U.S. Department of Health and Human Services, *Dietary Guidelines for Americans, 2010,* 7th ed. (Washington, DC: Government Printing Office, 2010), 12, https://health.gov/dietaryguidelines/dga2010/DietaryGuide lines2010.pdf.

128 **"veterinarians would not feed it":** Walter Willett, interview with the author, August 14, 2017. When Willett made this statement he was referring to the generally low quality of all carbohydrates in the American diet, not just wheat. But since wheat comprises the bulk of our carbohydrate intake I've made this small elision.

129 **"overall better alignment":** For the full investigation, see Sonia M. Grandi and Caroline Franck, "Agricultural Subsidies: Are They a Contributing Factor to the American Obesity Epidemic?," *JAMA Internal Medicine*172, no. 22, (2012): 1754–55.

129 **less than $1 billion:** "Overview of NOAA Fisheries' Budgets for Fiscal Years 2014 & 2015," a presentation to fisheries' stakeholders, NOAA Fisheries, national conference call and webinar, March 19, 2014, www.nmfs.noaa.gov/mb/budget/noaafisheries2014_2015budget.pdf. NOAA budget cuts are part of an overall 16 percent budget cut to the Department of Commerce, which oversees NOAA's fisheries and weather divisions. As *The Washington Post* reported in March 2017, "The Commerce cuts would eliminate $250 million in coastal research programs that prepare communities for rising seas and worsening storms, including the popular $73 million Sea Grant program, which works with universities in 33 states." Chris Mooney, "Proposed Budget for Commerce Would Cut Funds for NOAA," *The Washington Post,* March 16, 2017, www .washing tonpost.com/business/economy/proposed-budget-for-commerce-would-cut-funds-for -noaa/2017/03/15/6c93d864-09ad-11e7-93dc-00f9bdd74ed1_story.html?utm_term =.b6b65ecf1f00.

129 **cost of fruits and vegetables:** The relative price rises for fruits and vegetables and fats and oils can be found in Grandi and Franck, "Agricultural Subsidies," 1754. Similar price divergences are seen in emerging economies; a recent report of food prices in Brazil, Mexico, China, and South Korea found that fruits and vegetable prices increased by 91 percent while processed foods *declined* by 20 percent. Steve Wiggins and Sharada Keats, "The Rising Cost of a Healthy Diet: Changing Relative Prices of Foods in High-Income and Emerging Economies," Overseas Development Institute (ODI), May 2015, www.odi.org/rising-cost-healthy-diet. For an overall discussion of the low cost of high-energy diets versus the high cost of high-nutrient diets, see Nicole Darmon and Adam Drewnowski, "Contribution of Food Prices and Diet Cost to Socioeconomic Disparities in Diet Quality and Health: A Systematic Review and Analysis," *Nutrition Reviews* 73, no. 10 (October 2015): 643–60, www.ncbi.nlm.nih.gov/pmc/articles/PMC4586446/.

129 **"promiscuous and indiscriminate":** Dr. William Lands, interview with the author, May 17, 2017.

130 **"Obesity is associated":** Jørn Dyerberg and Richard Passwater, *The Missing Wellness Factors— EPA and DHA: The Most Important Nutrients Since Vitamins?* (Laguna Beach, CA: Basic Health Publications, 2012), 206. It is important to note here that research into the omega-3 effect on ameliorating type 2 diabetes is inconclusive. Studies have yielded conflicting results regarding which cholesterols are raised (in some cases "bad," or LDL, increases), whether insulin resistance is reduced, and which sources (fish, nuts, olive oil, supplements) of omega-3s might be helpful or might increase risks. See L. Azadbakht, M. H. Rouhani, and P. J. Surkan, "Omega-3 Fatty Acids, Insulin Resistance and Type 2 Diabetes," *Journal of Research in Medical Sciences* 16, no. 10 (October 2011): 1259–60. And for the explanation of how fat cells trigger an immune response that causes inflammation, see Methodist Hospital, Houston, "Obesity Makes Fat Cells Act Like They're Infected," *ScienceDaily,* March 5, 2013, www.sciencedaily.com/releases/2013/03/130305145 145.htm.

131 **the state of New Jersey:** The Gulf of Mexico dead zone reached the record-breaking size of 8,776 square miles, as reported by NOAA. New Jersey is 8,771 square miles, including water area. "Gulf of Mexico 'Dead Zone' Is the Largest Ever Measured," NOAA, August 2, 2017, www .noaa.gov/media-release/gulf-of-mexico-dead-zone-is-largest-ever-measured.

132 **1.7 million tons per year:** I originally published these facts about dead zones and of the connections between agriculture, fertilizer, the Mississippi, and the Gulf dead zone in Paul Greenberg, "A River Runs Through It," *American Prospect,* May 22, 2013.

133 **ocean's seemingly endless gifts:** Ibid., 2.

133 **dead zones now affect:** Robert J. Diaz and Rutger Rosenberg, "Spreading Dead Zones and Consequences for Marine Ecosystems," *Science* 321, no. 5891 (August 15, 2008): 926–29. For a map that shows where these global dead zones exist, see "Dead Zones," Virginia Institute of Marine Science, www.vims.edu/research/topics/dead_zones/index.php.

133 **corn and soybean farmer:** My visit with Brian Hicks and his story appear throughout Greenberg, "A River Runs Through It."

134 **nearly two Californias:** Total estimated corn acreage in 2017 was 90.9 million acres. Total estimated soy acreage in 2017 was 89.5 million acres. "Acreage," U.S. Department of Agriculture (USDA), ISSN: 1949-1522, June 30, 2017, https://usda.mannlib.cornell.edu/usda/current /Acre/Acre-06-30-2017.pdf. The total surface area of California is 155,779 square miles, which equals 99,698,560 acres. It should be noted, however, that farmers often rotate corn and soy in succession on the same piece of land.

134 **Jeff Strock, a professor:** Greenberg, "A River Runs Through It," 7.

135 **something like 30 percent:** Fertilizer cost varies depending on whether farmers are growing corn only, corn and soy, or more diverse systems. A representative chart for production in Iowa can be found from Iowa State's agriculture extension: "Estimated Costs of Crop Production in Iowa," Ag Decision Maker, Iowa State University, File A1-20, January 2017, www.extension .iastate.edu/agdm/crops/pdf/a1-20.pdf.

135 **This system is called tiling:** Greenberg, "A River Runs Through It," 7.

135 **forty-eight million acres:** "Conservation," 2012 Census of Agriculture, USDA, July 2014, 2, www.agcensus.usda.gov/Publications/2012/Online_Resources/Highlights/Conservation /Highlights_Conservation.pdf.

135 **the city of Des Moines:** The information about drinking water health issues, expenses, and pollution in the waters from agricultural fertilizer runoff in Des Moines, Iowa, is from Bill Stowe, interview with the author, October 18, 2017. Stowe is the Des Moines Water Works CEO and general manager and a fifth-generation native Iowan.

135 **blue baby syndrome:** "Nutrient Pollution. The Effects—Human Health," EPA, www.epa .gov/nutrientpollution/effects-human-health.

136 **"Look at the culverts":** Paul Greenberg, "How Your Diet Contributes to Water Pollution," *Eating Well,* July/August 2017, www.eatingwell.com/article/290358/how-your-diet-contributes-to-wa ter-pollution/.

136 **Toledo's municipal water supply:** Jugal K. Patel and Yuliya Parshina-Kottas, "Miles of Algae Covering Lake Erie," *The New York Times,* October 3, 2017, www.nytimes.com/interactive/2017 /10/03/science/earth/lake-erie.html.

136 **In China, beef consumption:** S. Anderson et al., *Chinese Beef Consumption Trends: Implications for Future Trading Partners,* Kansas State University, Department of Agricultural Economics, April 2011.

137 **eating more land food meat:** Tom Levitt, "China Facing Bigger Dietary Health Crisis Than the U.S.," *Chinadialogue,* July 4, 2014.

137 **200 percent higher:** Historical prices for commodity crops can be tracked with this tool presenting average U.S. farm prices from 1960 to the present: Darrel L. Good and Ping Li, "US Average Farm Price Received Database Tool," Farmdoc, University of Illinois, www.farmdoc .illinois.edu/manage/uspricehistory/us_price_history.html.

138 **the 1985 farm bill:** Greenberg, "A River Runs Through It," 6–7.

138 **the fastest destruction of grasslands:** See Christopher K. Wright and Michael C. Wimberly, "Recent Land Use Change in the Western Corn Belt Threatens Grasslands and Wetlands," *PNAS* 110, no. 10 (March 5, 2013): 4134–39.

140 **Chief among those critics:** Ibid., 9–10.

141 **A corn-stuffed rumen:** Pollan, "Power Steer."

142 **"Grain is fine"**: Tamar Haspel, "Is Grass-Fed Beef Really Better for You, the Animal and the Planet?," *The Washington Post*, February 23, 2015, www.washingtonpost.com/lifestyle/food /is-grass-fed-beef-really-better-for-you-the-animal-and-the-planet/2015/02/23/92733524 -b6d1-11e4-9423-f3d0a1ec335c_story.html?utm_term=.c694f5739ae7.

142 **five hundred million tons**: Julie Janovsky, "Industrial Animal Agriculture: A Broken System," PEW Charitable Trusts, June 2013, www.pewtrusts.org/~/media/assets/2011/07/19/pewindus trialanimalagriculturebrokensystemjuly2011.pdf.

142 **euphemistically calls lagoons**: Bill Field, "Beware of On-Farm Manure Storage Hazards," Rural Health and Safety Guide, Purdue University, S-82, www.extension.purdue.edu/extmedia /S/S-82.html.

143 **With the boat secured**: I first visited Paul Hartfield in the early spring of 2012 and over the years have interviewed him to discuss everything from dead zones to invasive Asian carp (which, he insists, are delicious). Some of these conversations with Hartfield were published in Greenberg, "A River Runs Through It," 11–14.

144 **River shrimp, Hartfield learned**: This is backed up by the literature of the time. A funny little pamphlet in the Historic New Orleans Collection called *Delphine the Little Shrimp Girl. A Story Intensified by Fate's Miraculous Doings* tells of a river girl's father who "pulled his shrimp bags out of the Mississippi river where they had been all night hanging from the levee in the high water to find he had quite a catch." Later her mother instructs her in a mix of Cajun and English, "Delphine ma fille, teck dis baskit of swimps down de coas, an sell heem, sell heem fo five cent de can." Martha Ellis Kenner, *Delphine the Little Shrimp Girl. A Story Intensified by Fate's Miraculous Doings* (self-published, 1923). Document available in the Historic New Orleans Collection, New Orleans, LA.

145 **Huck Finn a liar**: Huck reports in *Huckleberry Finn* that "about the first thing we done was to bait one of the big hooks with a skinned rabbit and set it to catch a cat-fish that was as big as a man, being six foot two inches long, and weighed over two hundred pounds. We couldn't handle him." Mark Twain, *Huckleberry Finn* (New York: Charles Webster & Company, 1885), 82.

146 **"faster and shorter"**: The reengineering of the Mississippi River is detailed in: John Barry, *Rising Tide: The Great Mississippi Flood of 1927 and How It Changed America* (New York: Simon & Schuster, 1997).

147 **In early New England**: Ted Steinberg, *Nature Incorporated: Industrialization and the Waters of New England* (Amherst: University of Massachusetts Press, 1994).

152 **used to make automobile fuel**: Jonathan Foley, "It's Time to Rethink America's Corn System," *Scientific American*, March 5, 2013, www.scientificamerican.com/article/time -to-rethink-corn/.

152 **ethanol production grew**: Tristan R. Brown, "Corn Ethanol: The Rise and Fall of a Political Force," *U.S. News & World Report*, February 3, 2016, www.usnews.com/news/articles/2016 -02-03/corn-ethanol-the-rise-and-fall-of-a-political-force.

152 **"Do we produce a product that is good?"**: Greenberg, "A River Runs Through It," 6.

152 **A review of a host of studies**: Brent D. Yacobucci and Randy Schnepf, "Ethanol and Biofuels: Agriculture, Infrastructure, and Market Constraints Related to Expanded Production," CRS Report for Congress, Order Code RL33928, March 16, 2007: 6–7, https://alternativeenergy .procon.org/sourcefiles/CRSreportEthanol2007.pdf.

153 **algae farmer Isaac Berzin**: Isaac Berzin, interview with the author, July 14, 2016.

155 **The "middleman" of the horse**: Mallory Warner, "How Horses Helped Cure Diphtheria," *Smithsonian*, August 15, 2013, http://americanhistory.si.edu/blog/2013/08/how-horses-helped -cure-diphtheria.html.

157 **"These algae are 40 percent"**: Various studies report *Nannochloropsis* sp. as having protein content as 30 percent or greater of organic content or dry weight. See Peter Coutteau, "Nutritional Value of Micro-algae," in P. Lavens and P. Sorgeloos, eds., "Manual on the Production and Use of Live Food for Aquaculture," *FAO Fisheries Technical Paper*, no. 361 (Rome: FAO, 1996): 31, and J. Fábregas et al., "The Cell Composition of *Nannochloropsis* sp. Changes Under Different Irradiances in Semicontinuous Culture," *World Journal of Microbiology and Biotechnology* 20, no. 1 (February 2004): 31–35.

CHAPTER SIX: AT THE BOTTOM OF IT ALL

162 **"Causabon's Key to All Mythologies":** Michael Pollan, correspondence with the author, May 10, 2017. "The Key to All Mythologies" is a book the fictional character Edward Causabon is writing in George Eliot's *Middlemarch.* Its author, a cleric of limited intellectual means, believes that his unwritten book will one day reveal that "all the mythical systems or erratic mythical fragments in the world were corruptions of a tradition originally revealed." His life's plan is to condense his "voluminous still-accumulating notes" into a set of volumes "like the earlier vintage of Hippo-cratic books, to fit on a little shelf." This great unifying treatise is never completed and his widow, Dorothea Brooke, discovers after her husband's death that the work is unpublishable.

163 **since the Industrial Revolution:** *World Ocean Review* puts it this way: "The ocean, with around 38,000 gigatons (Gt) of carbon (1 gigaton = 1 billion tons), contains 16 times as much carbon as the terrestrial biosphere, that is all plant and the underlying soils on our planet, and around 60 times as much as the pre-industrial atmosphere, i.e., before humans began to burn coal, oil and gas. At that time the carbon content of the atmosphere was only around 600 gigatons of carbon. The ocean is therefore the greatest of the carbon reservoirs, and essentially determines the atmo-spheric CO_2 content." "The Oceans—The Largest CO_2-Reservoir," *World Ocean Review,* http://worldoceanreview.com/en/wor-1/ocean-chemistry/co2-reservoir/. It should be noted, however, that there is a price to storage. The excess CO_2 can lead to a lowering of ocean pH, a phenomenon known as ocean acidification, and this buildup of CO_2 in deep, cold Antarctic waters can prevent krill larvae from developing or even stop the eggs from hatching. See S. Kawaguchi, et al., "Risk Maps for Antarctic Krill Under Projected Southern Ocean Acidification," *Nature Climate Change* 3 (2013): 843–47.

163 **map of Antarctica:** Sovereignty explains much of the time zone apportionment in Antarctica, though time in a large chunk of the White Continent is also governed by something called coor-dinated universal time, which is the principal time used for setting clocks and time worldwide. It is close to Greenwich mean time but, since the scientific community does not officially define Greenwich mean time, it is its own standard, within about 1 second of mean solar time at 0° lon-gitude. And, no, there is no daylight savings time with coordinated universal time. T. W., "What's the Time in Antarctica?," *Economist,* October 8, 2013, www.economist.com/blogs/economist -explains/2013/10/economist-explains-3.

165 **Norwegian vessel** *Saga Sea:* The *Saga Sea* was sighted that day at latitude 64.069 south, longitude 61.16 west.

166 **500 million metric tons:** CCAMLR, the international regulating commission overseeing the Antarctic fisheries, reports an estimated krill biomass of 379 million metric tons. This figure was arrived at in 2008 and published by A. Atkinson et al., "A Re-appraisal of the Total Biomass and Annual Production of Antarctic Krill," *Deep-Sea Research I* 56 (2009): 727–40.

166 **weight of** *all* **the fish:** The Food and Agriculture Organization of the United Nations generally places the legal catch at 80–90 million metric tons. Recently some researchers, in particular Dr. Daniel Pauly and other members of Sea Around Us at the University of British Columbia, have called into question that figure and suggest that if the illegal catch is included the number is more like 110 million metric tons. "Catches by Taxon in the Global Ocean," D. Pauly and D. Zeller, eds., *Catch Reconstruction: Concepts, Methods and Data Sources,* online publication (2015), Sea Around Us (www.seaaroundus.org), www.seaaroundus.org/data/#/global?chart=catch-chart& dimension=taxon&measure=tonnage&limit=10.

166 **Norwegian company called Aker BioMarine:** Norway is the major harvester of Antarctic krill and Aker BioMarine is the sole Norwegian fishing and biotech company catching krill in Antarc-tic waters. CCAMLR reports Norway as taking 58 percent of the catch, followed by the Republic of Korea (19 percent) and China (10 percent). "Krill—Biology, Ecology and Fishing," CCAMLR, www.ccamlr.org/en/fisheries/krill-%E2%80%93-biology-ecology-and-fishing.

167 **Cold War paranoias:** Peter J. Beck, *The International Politics of Antarctica* (London: Routledge Revivals, 2014), 52.

167 **"should leave a desert":** Yulia V. Ivashchenko and Phillip J. Clapham, "Too Much Is Never Enough: The Cautionary Tale of Soviet Illegal Whaling," *Marine Fisheries Review* 7, no. 1–2 (June 2014): 1.

167 **"whose main task":** Oleg Senetsky, "Statement by Soviet Fishing Inspector About Soviet Fisher-ies in the Southern Ocean," unpublished correspondence with Greenpeace Australia, August 1991 from the archive of the Antarctic krill researcher Dr. Stephen Nicol. Senetsky was head of

Marine Conventional Fisheries Inspection in Tallinn, Estonia, when he sent his letter to Greenpeace and other conservation groups in Australia to alert the world to the fact that Soviet officials were disregarding CCAMLR agreements and not reporting the full scope of their krill and icefish fishery.

168 "the U.S.S.R.'s desire": Ivashchenko and Clapham, "Too Much Is Never Enough," 1.

168 into those icy waters: Cassandra Brooks, email to the author, November 14, 2017. Professor Brooks wrote that "the Soviets had these huge fishing fleets with nowhere to go once UNCLOS was signed and 200 nautical mile exclusive economic zones came into being. They harvested finfish and krill in Antarctica not because these were ideal food, but because there was a lot of fish and very few fishing [there] at the time. The Russians at CCAMLR told me though that the fishery was highly subsidized, which is why the Russians largely dropped out after the fall of the USSR. And they also told me that the krill paste was terrible to eat."

168 large amounts of fluoride: Fluoride is contained in the shells, or exoskeletons, of krill and unless krill are immediately peeled, boiled, or frozen to lower than -30°C, the fluoride leaches into their tissues, making the flesh toxic to humans and land animals. Stephen Nicol, "Development of the Krill Fishing Industry," in "Harvesting Krill: Ecological Impact, Assessment, Products & Markets," T. J. Pitcher and R. Chuenpagdee, eds., *Fisheries Centre Research Report* 3, no. 3 (1995): 35–38.

169 feeding it to mink: There is scant record of the Soviet intent with respect to krill. A ghost of a reference is G. G. Besedina and N. S. Perel'dik, "Feeding of Krill (*Euphausia superba*) Paste to Female Minks," collection of scientific works—research institute of fur farming and rabbit breeding (USSR), AGRIS, FAO (1985), http://agris.fao.org/agris-search/search.do?recordID=SU8743970.

169 International Geophysical Year: It was truly an international event—sixty-seven countries participated in collaborative studies of the earth and atmosphere over a year and a half, with particular attention given to Antarctica. "The International Geophysical Year," National Academies, www.nas.edu/history/igy/.

170 (CCAMLR) wrote a founding charter: Background on the treaty, which is commonly pronounced "camel-r," can be found at: "About CCAMLR, History," CCAMLR, www.ccamlr.org /en/organisation/history.

170 cannot disturb wildlife: For the history and development of the CCAMLR's governance and the Antarctic Treaty, see "About CCAMLR, History of the Convention," CCAMLR, www.ccamlr .org/en/organisation/history-convention.

170 device called an Eco-Harvester: S. Nicol, J. Foster, and S. Kawaguchi, "The Fishery for Antarctic Krill—Recent Developments," *Fish and Fisheries* 13, no. 1 (2011): 30–40, and Susan Moran, "Team Tracks a Food Supply at the End of the World," *The New York Times*, March 12, 2012, 3.

170 a "rational use" clause: For a discussion of the original intent of "rational use" and the more recent debates about its meaning and application, see J. Jacquet et al., "'Rational Use' in Antarctic Waters," *Marine Policy* 63 (2016): 28–34.

171 digesting themselves upon death: Nicol, "Development of the Krill Fishing Industry," 36.

172 "Krill provides very good": Xie Yu, "Country Steps Up Operations in Antarctica to Benefit from Krill Bonanza," *China Daily USA*, March 4, 2015, http://usa.chinadaily.com.cn/epaper/2015-03 /04/content_19716649.htm.

172 China has asserted: Stuart Leavenworth, "China Fishing Plan in Antarctica Alarms Scientists," McClatchy DC Bureau, March 19, 2015, www.mcclatchydc.com/news/nation-world/world /article24781990.html.

172 No human had: Cassandra M. Brooks, "Competing Values on the Antarctic High Seas: CCAMLR and the Challenge of Marine-Protected Areas," *Polar Journal* 3, no. 2 (2013): 277–300.

172 whales in historic numbers: Atkinson et al. calculated the estimated predator biomass consumption of krill as 128–470 million metric tons per year, with the greater number exceeding the estimated biomass of 379 milion tons. This consumption is currently supported by including estimated krill growth with estimated biomass, but if predation was to increase and growth decrease, demand could outpace supply. A. Atkinson et al, "A Re-appraisal of the Total Biomass and Annual Production of Antarctic Krill."

173 "wasp waist" ecosystem: A. Atkinson et al., "Sardine Cycles, Krill Declines, and Locust Plagues: Revisiting 'Wasp-Waist' Food Webs," *Trends in Ecology and Evolution* 26, no. 6 (June 2014): 309–16.

174 **smaller summer phytoplankton bloom:** P. D. Rozema et al., "Interannual Variability in Phytoplankton Biomass and Species Composition in Northern Marguerite Bay (West Antarctic Peninsula) Is Governed by Both Winter Sea Ice Cover and Summer Stratification," *Limnology and Oceanography* 62, no. 1 (2017): 235–52.

175 **Bob Jacobel, a glaciologist:** Robert W. Jacobel, professor of physics, St. Olaf College, interviews with the author, December 2015–January 2016.

181 **a new record sea ice low:** "Sea Ice Hits Record Lows," National Snow and Ice Data Center (NSIDC), December 6, 2016, http://nsidc.org/arcticseaicenews/2016/12/arctic-and-antarctic-at -record -low-levels/.

181 **present krill habitat:** Andrea Thompson, "Krill Are Disappearing from Antarctic Waters," *Climate Central*, August 29, 2016, www.scientificamerican.com/article/krill-are-disappearing -from-antarctic-waters/, and "Climate Change Could Cause Major Decline in Antarctic Krill Habitat by 2100," American Geophysical Union, August 16, 2016, https://news.agu.org/press -release/climate-change-could-cause-major-decline-in-antarctic-krill-habitat-by-2100/.

182 **"pyramiding" his dogs:** Walter Sullivan, "The South Pole Fifty Years Later," *Arctic* 15, no. 3 (1962): 175–78.

182 **the global ocean is acidifying:** Before our current era, the last big carbon injection into the oceans was during the Paleocene-Eocene interval at fifty-six million years ago. Bärbel Hönisch et al., in "The Geological Record of Ocean Acidification," reach a chilling conclusion: "The current rate of (mainly fossil fuel) CO_2 release stands out as capable of driving a combination and magnitude of ocean geochemical changes potentially unparalleled in at least the last 300 million years of Earth history, raising the possibility that we are entering an unknown territory of marine ecosystem change." Bärbel Hönisch et al., "The Geological Record of Ocean Acidification," *Science* 335 (2012): 1058–63.

182 **some of the largest declines:** D. G. Boyce et al., "Estimating Global Chlorophyll Changes over the Past Century," *Progress in Oceanography* 122 (2014): 163–73.

183 **a "methane burp":** Alanna Mitchell, *Seasick: Ocean Change and the Extinction of Life on Earth* (Chicago: University of Chicago Press, 2009), 98–99.

184 **"The room just erupted":** The attendee to the meeting who said these words was the writer, photographer, filmmaker, and conservationist John Weller. His book *The Last Ocean: Antarctica's Ross Sea Project: Saving the Most Pristine Ecosystem on Earth* (New York: Rizzoli, 2013) documents in words and photographs much of the struggle to protect the Ross Sea. Conversation with the author, July 2016.

CHAPTER SEVEN: TOWARD AN OMEGA-3 WORLD

188 **methane and nitrous oxide:** H. Steinfeld et al., *Livestock's Long Shadow: Environmental Issues and Options* (Rome: FAO, 2006), 82–83.

188 **corn occupies the lion's share:** USDA, "Acreage," 1.

188 **service of producing carbohydrates:** As with most dietary studies, the researcher must rely on association studies rather than more rigorous randomized controlled trials. But large association studies do carry weight. In 2017 the Prospective Urban Rural Epidemiology (PURE) study synthesized dietary surveys from more than 135,000 people across five continents and found that a diet that includes moderate intake of fat, high amounts of fruits and vegetables and avoidance of high carbohydrates is associated with lower risk of death. V. Miller et al., "Fruit, Vegetable, and Legume Intake, and Cardiovascular Disease and Deaths in 18 Countries: A Prospective Cohort Study," *Lancet* 390 (November 4, 2017): 2037–49, www.thelancet.com/pdfs/journals /lancet/PIIS0140-6736(17)32253-5.pdf.

189 **Much of our cooking oil:** Raj Patel, *Stuffed and Starved: The Hidden Battle for the World Food System* (Brooklyn, NY: Melville House, 2012), 176.

189 **draining of swampy, marginal areas:** Keith Ouchley, interview with the author, March 3, 2013. The cutting of bottomland forest and the conversion of wetlands to soy production was relayed to me during a visit to bottomland forest in southern Mississippi and northern Louisiana with Ouchley, who is the Mississippi state director of the Nature Conservancy. Further information about the conversion of bottomland forest to soy can be found in Herbert S. Sternitzke and Joe F. Christopher, "Land Clearing in the Lower Mississippi Valley," *Southeastern Geographer* 10, no. 1 (April, 1970): 63–66.

189 **U.S. Department of Agriculture recommends:** Arlin Wasserman, conversation with the author, June 30, 2016. Protein recommendations vary depending on the subject's weight, age, gender, and

level of activity. The range presented were the averages as interpreted by Wasserman. The USDA offers an online calculator to determine the appropriate amount of protein for a given individual at: "Interactive DRI for Health Care Professionals," Food and Nutrition Information Center, USDA, www.nal.usda.gov/fnic/interactiveDRI/.

190 **whatever protein it cannot use:** Michael Tlusty and Peter Tyedmers, "Eat Too Much Protein, Piss Away Sustainability," Triple Pundit, November 23, 2015, www.triplepundit.com/2015/11/eat-much-protein-piss-away-sustainability/.

190 **impending "protein deficit":** The protein deficit is a common theme within world food forums. Just one example can be found here: "The Protein Challenge 2040," Forum for the Future, www.forumforthefuture.org/project/protein-challenge-2040/overview.

190 **nine billion humans:** As of April 2017, the United Nations estimated the world population at seven and a half billion and predicts an increase to nine billion by 2050.

191 **Gaines is a marine ecologist:** Steve Gaines, interview with the author, March 24, 2017.

191 **the earth's freshwater:** "Thirsty Food: Fueling Agriculture to Fuel Humans," *National Geographic,* http://environment.nationalgeographic.com/environment/freshwater/food/.

191 **the world's energy:** "'Energy-Smart' Agriculture Needed to Escape Fossil Fuel Trap," FAO, November 29, 2011, www.fao.org/news/story/en/item/95161/icode/.

191 **the planet's arable land:** Jelle Bruinsma, ed., *World Agriculture: Towards 2015/2030. An FAO Perspective* (London: Earthscan Publications, 2003), 127.

192 **life spans of subjects:** For more nuanced details of the diet/environment/health overlap, including regional complexities of diet, the effects of various methods of food production on greenhouse gas emissions and land use, and income influence on diet choices, see David Tilman and Michael Clark, "Global Diets Link Environmental Sustainability and Human Health," *Nature* 515 (November 27, 2014): 518–22.

195 **Jackson's crops would primarily feed:** My write-up of Wes Jackson's ideas for developing Kernza and perennial crops originally appeared in Greenberg, "A River Runs Through It," *American Prospect,* May 22, 2013, 9.

196 **$15 billion in farm subsidies:** "USDA FY 2018 Budget Summary," USDA, page 14, Table FFAS-6, line for Subtotal, Commodity Payments, and page 19, Table FFAS-11, line for Total Mandatory, www.obpa.usda.gov/budsum/fy18budsum.pdf.

196 **plant breeder Lee DeHaan:** Lee DeHaan, interview with the author, April 13, 2017, and follow-up email, October 16, 2017.

197 **Guy Choiniere in Highgate Center:** This portrayal of Guy Choiniere's farm is drawn from my earlier article, Greenberg, "How Your Diet Contributes to Water Pollution" *Eating Well Magazine,* May/June, 2017.

199 **Currently around 40 percent:** Foley, "It's Time to Rethink America's Corn System," *Scientific American,* March 5, 2013, www.scientificamerican.com/article/time-to-rethink-corn.

200 **Roscoe Wind Farm:** Cliff Etheridge, Abilene, Texas, site visit and interview with the author, January 24, 2010. Additional background on Etheridge's wind projects in Texas can be found at "Fort Worth Telegram—Rancher's Windfall—More West Texas Landowners Are Signing Deals with Wind-Farm Developers," Cielo Wind Power via *Fort Worth Star-Telegram,* record number 1950956, January 29, 2006, www.cielowind.com/news/articles/fort-worth-telegram-ranchers-windfall; and "Airtricity Finalizes Largest Wind Project to Date," Business Wire, May 15, 2007, www.businesswire.com/news/home/20070515006023/en/Airtricity-Finalizes-Largest-Wind-Project-Date.

201 **Catching wild fish:** Robert W. R. Parker and P. H. Tyedmers, "Fuel Consumption of Global Fishing Fleets: Current Understanding and Knowledge Gaps," *Fish and Fisheries* 16 (2015): 684–96. The authors present a comparison of fisheries to other protein production based on the carbon footprint prior to processing and transport—the most fuel-efficient fisheries use less than 3 kilograms of CO_2 per kilogram of live weight, whereas beef production requires an estimated 10 kilograms of CO_2 per kilogram of cattle.

202 **fined Trident Seafood:** See the consent decree Trident entered into with the EPA for more information. Frederick Phillips, *"United States of America, Plaintiff vs. TRIDENT SEAFOODS CORPORATION, Defendant. Consent Decree,"* Environment and Natural Resources Division, United States Department of Justice, August 2011, www.epa.gov/sites/production/files/documents/trident-cd.pdf.

203 **manufacturer named Sandro Lane:** Sandro Lane, interview with the author, June 9, 2016. For more information on Alaska Protein Recovery and Pure Alaska Omega Salmon Oil, see www.alaskaproteinrecovery.com/home and www.purealaskaomega.com/our-story/.

204 **The Norwegian company BioMar:** Statistics on BioMar and other feed company ingredient portfolios were provided by Vidar Gunderson of BioMar, email to the author, October 27, 2017, who used the following report as reference for his comments: "Sustainability Report 2016," BioMar Group, www.biomar.com/globalassets/.global/blocks-content—images-_en/c -sustainability-_en/5.-guidelines—reporting-_en/biomar-gri-report_2016_web.pdf.

204 **eating land animal flesh:** Rick Barrows, interview with the author, March 25, 2016.

206 **its own economy of scale:** Since I spoke with Barrows in the summer of 2016 there have been numerous developments in producing fish-free feed. A competition called the F3 Challenge sponsored by the University of Arizona, the University of Massachusetts Boston, Synbiobeta, the Anthropocene Institute, and the World Bank has spurred competitions for a fish-free feed and a fish-free "fish oil": "F3 Fish Oil Challenge," https://f3challenge.org/. And now Coppens International has a line of feed called NeoGreen that has an algae-derived fish oil replacer called ForPlus. "Coppens International Unveils Breakthrough Aquatic Feed Innovations for 2017," press release, Alltech, January 17, 2017, www.alltech.com/news/news-articles/2017/01/17/coppens -international-unveils-breakthrough-aquatic-feed-innovations.

207 **rapeseed has a long history:** "Rapeseed," Agricultural Marketing Resource Center, www .agmrc.org/commodities-products/grains-oilseeds/rapeseed/.

207 **roughly 65 percent of feed:** From a Norwegian report on feed composition provided to me by Vidar Gunderson: T. Ytrestøyl et al., "Resource Accounting and Analysis of Feed Materials 2012: Final Report," Nofima, Report 51/2014, December 2014: 4, https://brage.bibsys.no/xmlui /bitstream/handle/11250/283694/Rapport51-2014.pdf?sequence=3&isAllowed=y.

208 **giant pile of maggots:** Greg Wanger, interview with the author, September 15, 2017.

208 **North Americans throw out:** Adam Chandler, "Why Americans Lead the World in Food Waste," *Atlantic*, July 15, 2016, www.theatlantic.com/business/archive/2016/07/american-food -waste/491513/.

209 **a quick calculation:** Greg Wanger, email to the author, October 25, 2017. Wanger's food-to-fly calculation, and his references were: "60 million tons of organic waste per year in North America (ibid). Take 15 to 20 percent of the 60 million tons - food conversion from the wet weight of organic matter to black soldier fly larvae (BSFL) = 12–15 million tons of BSFL/year. Food to larvae conversion: Haeree H. Park, "Black Soldier Fly Larvae Manual," *Student Showcase* 14, University of Massachusetts–Amherst (2016), 9, http://scholarworks.umass.edu/cgi/viewcontent.cgi?arti-cle=1015&context=sustainableumass_studentshowcase."

209 **Yeast can be grown:** According to Dr. Margareth Øverland of the Fakuletet for iovitenskap, Institutt for husdyrog akvakulturvitenskap, yeast can be grown on a substrate of lumber by-products. Bacteria can be produced on a plume of natural gas. Margareth Øverland, interview with the author, November 8, 2017.

210 **attention by Bren Smith:** This very condensed account of Smith's ocean farm is based on several site visits from 2011 to 2016. Smith is the owner of Thimble Island Oyster Co. in Long Island Sound.

211 **markedly lower methane emissions:** R. D. Kinley et al., "The Red Macroalgae Asparagopsis taxiformis Is a Potent Natural Antimethanogenic That Reduces Methane Production During In Vitro Fermentation with Rumen Fluid," *Animal Production Science* 56, no. 3 (2016): 282–89.

213 **founder of Pemaquid Mussel Farms:** Carter Newell's quotes and descriptions of his mussel farm first appeared in Paul Greenberg, "How Mussel Farming Could Help to Clean Fouled Waters," *Yale Environment* 360, May 9, 2013, http://e360.yale.edu/features/how_mussel_farming_could _help_to_clean_fouled_waters.

214 **Eva Galimany, a marine biologist:** Dr. Eva Galimany was originally quoted in Greenberg, "How Mussel Farming Could Help to Clean Fouled Waters."

214 **bivalves are far down:** In the National Fisheries Institute's annual report on the ten most consumed seafoods in America, the only bivalve that breaks into the top ten is clams. Americans consumed only about .33 pounds of clams per person in 2015 compared with 2.8 pounds of salmon and 2.3 pounds of tuna. Meanwhile, consumption of terrestrial animals was well over 100 pounds per capita. Cliff White, "NFI Lists America's Top 10 Favorite Seafood Species," SeafoodSource, October 31, 2016, www.seafoodsource.com/news/supply-trade/nfi-lists-america -s-top-10-favorite-seafood-species.

215 **high-quality protein:** Odd Lindahl, interview with the author, July 6, 2017. For more information on Dr. Lindahl's development of mussels as feed, visit the Musselfeed company website at Musselfeed.com. And for the research on the environmental benefits of mussel farming, see

O. Lindahl et al., "Improving Marine Water Quality by Mussel Farming: A Profitable Solution," *Ambio* 34, no. 2 (March 2005): 131–38.

215 **Offshore wind is both stronger:** "Are Wind Speeds the Same over Land as They Are over the Ocean?," National Data Buoy Center, NOAA, www.ndbc.noaa.gov/educate/windspeed_ans.shtml.

216 **"When we analyzed":** Willett Kempton, in visit to Kempton's lab and interview with the author, January 28, 2010. For more information on resource size and comparisons to regional end uses and all U.S. Atlantic petroleum, see W. Kempton et al., "Large CO_2 Reductions via Offshore Wind Power Matched to Inherent Storage in Energy End-Uses," *Geophysical Research Letters* 34, no. 2 (January 2007), doi:10.1029/2006GL028016.

216 **30 percent of our energy:** "Electricity Explained: Electricity in the United States," U.S. Energy Information Adminstration (EIA), www.eia.gov/energyexplained/index.cfm?page=electricity _in_the_united_states.

216 **the world's anthropogenic mercury:** "Mercury Emissions: The Global Context," EPA, www .epa.gov/international-cooperation/mercury-emissions-global-context; and AMAP/UNEP, "Global Mercury Modelling: Update of Modelling Results in the Global Mercury Assessment 2013," Arctic Monitoring and Assessment Programme, Oslo, Norway/UNEP Chemicals Branch, 2015, https://wedocs.unep.org/bitstream/handle/20.500.11822/11440/Report-Model lingupdateoftheGMA2013.pdf.pdf?sequence=1&isAllowed=y.

217 **"this decrease parallels":** C. Lee et al., "Declining Mercury Concentrations in Bluefin Tuna Reflect Reduction Emissions to the North Atlantic Ocean," *Environmental Science and Tecchnology* 50, no. 23 (2016): 12825–30, http://pubs.acs.org/doi/abs/10.1021/acs.est.6b04328.

217 **The element selenium:** The selenium argument is debated most recently in this article: Darryl Fears, "Fish Fight: Scientists Battle over the True Harm of Mercury in Tuna," *The Washington Post,* March 4, 2017, www.washingtonpost.com/national/health-science/fish-fight-scientists-battle -over-the-true-harm-of-mercury-in-tuna/2017/03/04/2210fe74-f2d4-11e6-8d72 -263470bf0401_story.html?utm_term=.9063f392c892.

217 **An offshore wind farm:** B. H. Buck et al., "The German Case Study: Pioneer Projects of Aquaculture-Wind Farm Multi-Uses," in *Aquaculture Perspective of Multi-Use Sites in the Open Ocean: The Untapped Potential for Marine Resources in the Anthropocene,* B. Buck and R. Langan, eds. (Cham, Switzerland: Springer, 2017), 253–354.

218 **Aquaculture and harmful algal bloom:** Dr. Jack Rensel was originally quoted in Paul Greenberg, "Nations Have Carved Up the Ocean. Now What?," *Conservation,* University of Washington, March 14, 2014, www.conservationmagazine.org/2014/03/aquaculture-in -us-federal-waters/. Expansion on the topic occurred in Dr. Rensel, email to the author, October 19, 2017.

CONCLUSION

221 **temperature for September 2017:** "State of the Climate: National Climate Report for September 2017," NOAA National Centers for Environmental Information, published online October 2017, www.ncdc.noaa.gov/sotc/national/201709.

222 **Omega Protein, had morphed:** Franklin, *The Most Important Fish in the Sea: Menhaden and America* (Washington, DC: Island Press, 2009), 206–8.

222 **three hundred million fish:** The reduction industry caught 137,400 metric tons of menhaden in 2016. Conservatively multiplying the annual reduction catch by 2,200 pounds, with an assumption that fish averaged one pound (on the high side for menhaden's adult weight), gives a conservative estimate of 300 million fish. Since Omega Protein is the primary reduction company fishing menhaden, we can assume that the bulk of those fish were caught by that company. It should be noted that the reduction industry's 2016 catch is far below the historical high of 1.5 billion fish in 1955. "Atlantic Menhaden," Atlantic States Marine Fisheries Commission, Fisheries Management, www.asmfc.org/species/atlantic-menhaden.

222 **a changed sea:** Safina's article on the menhaden's return to abundance and continued threats from fishing is: Carl Safina, "The Great East Coast Return to Abundance—Your Help Needed," Ocean Views, *National Geographic,* September 4, 2017, https://voices.nationalgeographic.org /2017/09/04/the-great-east-coast-return-to-abundance-your-help-needed/.

223 **lowering of fishing pressure:** Professor Ray Hilborn at the University of Washington, who frequently disagrees with conclusions reached by the conservation community, wrote to me on hearing of the strong showing of menhaden in 2017, "It is clear there is no relationship between

spawning stock size and recruitment for Atlantic menhaden . . . so if the 'runs' are young fish then changing the harvest has had nothing to do with it." Ray Hillborn, email to the author, October 17, 2017.

223 **"A blind man can see":** Captain Paul Eidman, email to the author, October 16, 2017. His full email read: "Yes I believe that the increased size of the adult bunker schools in the NY/NJ bight are a direct result of our conservation efforts towards implementation of catch moderation regs. Compared to recent previous seasons all you have to do is use fall surf fishing alone as a barometer. The past two years of peanut bunker (young of year) runs down the beach have made for some phenomenal striped bass blitzes well within reach of the beach. A blind man can see the impact of catch limits with all the osprey, whales, dolphins, sharks, striped bass and blues feeding upon the resurgence of local bunker populations."

223 **I sat in:** The full transcript of the May 2015 menhaden meeting can be found at: "Proceedings of the Atlantic States Marine Fisheries Commission Atlantic Menhaden Management Board," Alexandria, VA (May 5, 2015): 1–50, www.asmfc.org/uploads/file/564b9744AtlMenhaden Board Proceedings_May2015.pdf.

224 **Council met again to debate:** Dave Mayfield, "Big Change for a Little Fish? Menhaden Board Says: Not So Fast," *Virginian-Pilot*, updated November 13, 2017, https://pilotonline.com/news /local/environment/big-change-for-a-little-fish-menhaden-board-says-not/article_fc438171 -2538-5548-b09a-7800ef605faf.html?__vfz=medium%3Dsharebar.

224 **ecosystem reference points:** Ben Landry, director of public affairs, Omega Protein Corporation, conversation with the author, December 15, 2017.

OMEGA IN THE KITCHEN

236 **tomato and anchovy sauce:** Marcella Hazan, *Essentials of Classic Italian Cooking* (New York: Alfred A. Knopf, 1992), 174.

247 **Glasmastarsill, or Glassblower's Herring:** This recipe was drawn from Hank Shaw, "Swedish Pickled Herring," Hunter Angler Gardener Cook, https://honest-food.net/swedish-pickled -herring/.

250 **Roulades of Antarctic Penguin Breast:** Gerald T. Cutland, *Fit for a FID Cookbook* (Base F: Wordie House, 1957).

Index

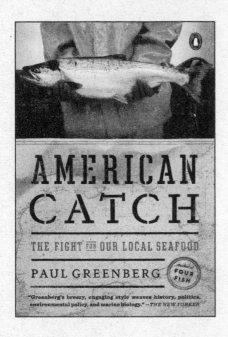

Four Fish

The Future of the Last Wild Food

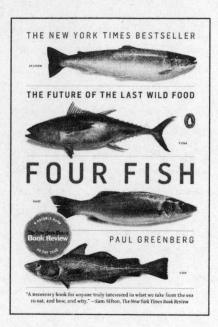

In *Four Fish*, Paul Greenberg reveals our damaged relationship with the ocean and its inhabitants. Just three decades ago, nearly everything we ate from the sea was wild. Today, rampant overfishing and an unprecedented biotech revolution have brought us to a point where wild and farmed fish occupy equal parts of a complex marketplace. *Four Fish* offers a way for us to move toward a future in which healthy and sustainable seafood is the rule rather than the exception.

"The engrossing story of the impact of history, geography, and politics on our seafood [and] a clear-eyed manifesto for the future of fish." *–Financial Times*

PENGUIN BOOKS